Fundamentals of Pap Test Cytology

By

Rana S. Hoda, MD, FIAC

Department of Pathology
Medical University of South Carolina
Charleston, SC

Syed A. Hoda, MD

Department of Pathology
Weill Medical College of Cornell University
and
New York Weill-Cornell Medical Center
New York, NY

Foreword by

Prabodh K. Gupta, MB, BS, MD, FIAC

Department of Pathology and Laboratory Medicine
University of Pennsylvania School of Medicine
and
Director of Cytopathology and Cytometry
University of Pennsylvania Health System
Philadelphia, PA

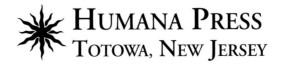

HUMANA PRESS
TOTOWA, NEW JERSEY

This publication is printed on acid-free paper. ∞
ANSI Z39.48-1984 (American Standards Institute) Permanence of Paper for Printed Library Materials.

Cover illustration: From Fig. 13.11 of Chapter 13 titled "Invasive Squamous Carcinoma."

Cover design by Donna Niethe.

Production Editor: Amy Thau

For additional copies, pricing for bulk purchases, and/or information about other Humana titles, contact Humana at the above address or at any of the following numbers: Tel.: 973-256-1699; Fax: 973-256-8314; E-mail: humana@humanapr.com, or visit our Website: http://humanapress.com

Photocopy Authorization Policy:

Authorization to photocopy items for internal or personal use, or the internal or personal use of specific clients, is granted by Humana Press Inc., provided that the base fee of US $25.00 per copy is paid directly to the Copyright Clearance Center at 222 Rosewood Drive, Danvers, MA 01923. For those organizations that have been granted a photocopy license from the CCC, a separate system of payment has been arranged and is acceptable to Humana Press Inc. The fee code for users of the Transactional Reporting Service is: [978-1-58829-768-6 • 1-58829-768-3/07 $30.00].

Printed in the United States of America. 10 9 8 7 6 5 4 3 2 1
eISBN:1-59745-276-9
Library of Congress Cataloging in Publication Data
Hoda, Rana S.
 Fundamentals of PAP test cytology / by Rana S. Hoda, Syed A. Hoda.
  p. ; cm.
 Includes bibliographical references and index.
 ISBN 1-58829-768-3 (alk. paper)
 1. Pap test. 2. Vaginal smears. 3. Cervix uteri--Cancer--Diagnosis. I. Hoda, Syed A. II. Title.
 [DNLM: 1. Vaginal Smears. 2. Cervix Uteri--cytology. 3. Cervix Uteri--pathology. 4. Uterine Cervical Diseases--diagnosis. WP 141 H687f 2007]
 RG107.5.P3H63 2007
 618.1'40757--dc22
                              2006017635

Dedication

To our parents, Atiqa and Shafiq Siddiqi, and Rabia and Qamar Hoda;
and to our to our son, Raza, the light of our lives.

Foreword

Over the past 50 years, cervical cancer detection by Papanicolaou smear examination has undergone a gradual evolution, but more recently, a revolution. Drs. Rana and Syed Hoda have positioned themselves at the forefront of this metamorphosis; the accurate, economical, and rapid detection procedure is now dubbed "the Pap test" for cervical cancer screening. During this time, many mysteries of cervical cancer have been unraveled. The mononuclears are the precancerous cells, and the toxins include human papilloma virus (HPV) as the major culprit. Papanicolaou's concept that "mononuclears reacted to the cancerous toxins in a way as to make them cytologically recognized" remains prophetic and true! Cervical specimens are collected in fluids instead of glass slides. Cells are processed utilizing propriety machines; morphological alterations are detected either manually or by morphometric techniques. Specimens are tested for the "toxins"-HPV. Changing times have required redefining the cytomorphological features and an accurate recognition of developing cervical cancer in all its variegates. The Bethesda System along with HPV type recognition has become the "standard of care."

Drs. Rana and Syed Hoda are highly respected in the pathology community. Their reputation as lucid, competent, objective, and elegant writers is well established. In *Fundamentals of Pap Test Cytology*, the Hoda's have provided a comprehensive review of the topic; it is timely and up to date. This book fills an important space in the gynecological cytopathology field. Authors will capitalize on their experience and concepts; succinct and relevant presentation is the linchpin of *Fundamentals of Pap Test Cytology*. It testifies to being a labor of love and patience. Drs. Rana and Syed Hoda need to be congratulated for providing this most timely publication. It provides all the information necessary to practice modern gynecological cytopathology. Their book will be valuable to the cytopathology community and help improve health care of all women.

Prabodh K. Gupta, MB, BS, MD, FIAC
Department of Pathology and Laboratory Medicine
University of Pennsylvania School of Medicine
Director of Cytopathology and Cytometry
University of Pennsylvania Health System
Philadelphia, PA

Preface

The "Pap" test (cervicovaginal cytology screening test) is currently the standard of care for screening for preneoplastic and neoplastic cervical diseases. The drastic decline in morbidity and mortality from cervical disease is directly attributable to this test. Although there are several exceptionally erudite cytopathology textbooks that discuss this test in great detail, clinically important information is often difficult to find, usually being buried under mountains of text. There is, to date, no concise textbook that deals with the basic practical issues regarding Pap tests.

Fundamentals of Pap Test Cytology is intended as a practical primer on the Pap test. The uniform layout and the selective use of bold text and tables are user-friendly, and intended to render finding specific information effortless. It is hoped that all involved in screening of the Pap test, including cytotechnologists and cytopathologists, as well as those in training, will reach for this primer first.

Fundamentals of Pap Test Cytology is lean enough to be easily read cover to cover within a reasonably short period of time. It is hoped that the reader will refer to this book often, or as the need arises, to learn more about the various cytopathological, technical, and clinical aspects of the Pap test. The book is also intended to help the reader readily understand the diagnostic implications of various lesions. Lastly, it is hoped that readers will find helpful information throughout these pages for taking various proficiency and licensing examinations.

Rana S. Hoda, MD, FIAC
Syed A. Hoda, MD

Acknowledgments

The authors concede their deep debt to Mr. James Nicholson of Medical University of South Carolina for his proficient and professional help with photomicroscopy, digital imaging and related techniques.

The support (in words and deeds) provided by the authors' respective departmental Chairpersons—Dr. Daniel Knowles (at Weill-Cornell) and Dr. Janice Lage (at Medical University of South Carolina)—is gratefully acknowledged.

The guidance, knowledge, and training imparted to the authors by their many beloved teachers including, in alphabetical order: Drs. Prabodh K. Gupta (who kindly wrote the Foreword to this work), Stephen Hajdu, Leopold Koss, Paul Peter Rosen, Richard J. Reed, and Juan Rosai, are treasured beyond words.

Contents

1

A Short Dictionary of the Pap Test

Acanthosis: thickening of the epithelium; a reactive and protective phenomenon.

Acidophilia: staining reaction: pink with eosin dyes; also known as eosinophilia.

Actinomyces: dark filamentous bacteria in clumps; common with intra-uterine device use.

Adequate Pap test: conventional smear with 8000–12,000 (and liquid-based preparations with ≥ 5000) well-preserved and well-visualized squamous cells.

Air-drying artifact: limits interpretation, affects the nucleus and the cytoplasm, imparts eosinophilia to the nucleus, usually accounts for a higher atypical squamous cells of unde-termined significance (ASC-US) rate; air-drying is uncommon in thin-layer preparations.

Alternaria: air-borne contaminant that looks like "snow shoes."

Amenorrhea: may be primary or secondary.

    Primary: patient has never menstruated; indicates a congenital defect.

    Secondary: cessation of menses; indicates pregnancy or ovarian failure.

Amorphous: without form or shape.

Amphophilia: cell with acidophilic and basophilic cytoplasmic staining.

Anaplasia: loss of differentiation, organization, and function in a tumor cell.

Anisocytosis: a notable variation in the size or the shape of cells.

Anisokaryosis: notable variation in the size or the shape of nuclei.

Anucleate squames: orangeophilic, large flat squamous cell devoid of a nucleus.

Apoptosis: programmed cell death—could be either physiological or pathological.

Arias–Stella reaction: endometrium and cervix in pregnancy, characterized by large cells with vacuolated cytoplasm, round nuclei, and a high nuclear-to-cytoplasmic (n:c) ratio.

ASC-H: atypical squamous cells cannot exclude high-grade squamous intra-epithelial lesion (HSIL); small squamous metaplastic, high n:c cells with slight hyperchromasia, and irreg-ularity of the nuclear membrane.

ASC-US: slight nuclear enlargement (two and a half to three times intermediate cell nuclei), hyperchromasia, membrane irregularity, and an increase in n:c.

Atrophic smears: characterized by dominance of parabasal cells.

Atrophic vaginitis: atrophy with inflammation and dirty granular background.

Atypia: any deviation from normal cellular morphology.

Atypical parakeratosis: two-dimensional fragments of slightly orangeophilic, miniature squa-mous cells with elongated, large, irregular, hyperchromatic nuclei, and mildly high n:c.

Atypical repair: loss of nuclear polarity, anisonucleosis, hyperchromasia with irregular chro-matin distribution, prominent and multiple nucleoli, mild membrane irregularities, single cells; mimics squamous-cell carcinoma.

Atypical squamous metaplasia: enlarged nuclei with a slightly irregular nuclear membrane, mild hyperchromasia, and high n:c; mimics HSIL.

Basophilia: also known as cyanophilia; stains blue or purple with basic dyes.

Binucleation: may be seen with ASC-US, human papillomavirus (HPV), or various infections.

From: *Fundamentals of Pap Test Cytology*
By: R. S. Hoda and S. A. Hoda © Humana Press Inc., Totowa, NJ

"Blue blobs:" degenerated parabasal cells characteristic of atrophy.

Brown artifact: "corn flakes," air-trapping under a cover slip—"brown cell" artifact.

Brush artifact: glandular crowding: aggressive sampling via endocervix brush; mimics adenocarcinoma *in situ* (AIS).

***Candida albicans*:** a variety of fungus encountered in the Pap test.

Caudate cell: tadpole-shaped cells; nucleus in the "head" is seen in keratinizing squamous-cell carcinoma.

Chlamydia trachomatis: obligatory intracellular bacteria, cytological changes are nondiagnostic; may be associated with follicular cervicitis.

"Clue cells:" tiny coccobacillary organisms covering squamous cells caused by a variety of microorganisms; interpreted as a *"shift in vaginal flora."*

Cytomegalovirus-infected cell: uncommon in Pap smears; cellular and nuclear enlargement, single large, round, intranuclear inclusion, a thin halo; small basophilic cytoplasmic inclusions.

Cockleburs: hematoidin crystals appear as cockleburs.

"Corn flaking:" air-trapping under a cover slip, also known as "brown cell" artifact.

Crowded cell index: one of the hormonal indices that indicates the ratio of clusters of more than four cells to single squamous cells.

Cyanophilia: also known as basophilia; stains blue or purple with basic dyes.

Cytolysis: usually with *lactobacilli* resulting in dissolution of cytoplasm of intermediate squamous cells leaving "bare nuclei," which may mimic benign-appearing endometrial cells.

Decidual cells: stromal cells with progesterone effect.

Degenerative changes: nuclear (e.g., smudged chromatin) or cytoplasmic (e.g., vacuoles).

Differentiation: the morphological and functional specialization of a cell.

Disordered honeycomb: AIS of the endocervix on thin-layer preparations.

Doderlein's bacilli: heterogeneous group of *lactobacilli*.

Dyskeratosis: keratinization of cells below the granular layer; premature.

Dyskaryosis: also known as dysplasia; generally not used in the United States.

Dysplasia: abnormal alteration of epithelia, characterized by increased primitive cells associated with variable surface maturation and abnormal differentiation.

Endometrial cells: small cells in three-dimensional clusters, nuclei are round and equal to size of intermediate cell nuclei.

Eosinophilia: the property of staining pink or red with eosin dye.

Eosinophilic index: one of the hormonal indices that indicates the percentage of mature superficial cells with eosinophilic cytoplasm among all other superficial and intermediate cells.

Epithelial "pearl:" concentric structure with keratinized cells; nuclei are retained.

Estrogenic effect: proportion of superficial cells reflect estrogenic effect.

"Exodus:" histiocytes + endometrial, epithelial, and stromal clusters representing a menstrual smear; common day 6–10 of the menstrual cycle.

"Feathering:" peripheral nuclear protrusion characteristic of AIS of the endocervix.

Ferning: arborizing a "palm leaf-like" pattern of mucus at ovulation.

Folded cell index: one of the hormonal indices that indicates the ratio of folded-to-nonfolded cytoplasm in mature squamous cells.

Folic acid deficiency: cytomegaly, nuclear enlargement, binucleation, chromatin, and cytoplasm are unchanged; mimics ASC-US.

Follicular cervicitis: lymphocytes and tingible-body histiocytes in a Pap smear are associated with *Chlamydia trachomatis* in approx 50% of cases.

Glandular grouping: usually three-dimensional; poorly defined cell borders.

Halo: vacuole around the nucleus is typically larger and optically clear in HPV-infected cells; a smaller halo is seen in *Trichomonas* infection and folic deficiency.

Hemosiderin and hematoidin: seen in conditions causing hemorrhage, such as the postpartum period.

Herpesvirus-infected cell: ground-glass nuclei; multinucleated cells with nuclear molding.

Histiocyte: cell with an ill-defined border, finely vacuolated cytoplasm, may have engulfed material in cytoplasm, and a pale, rounded, and reniform nucleus that is often eccentrically located.

"Hobnail" cell: characteristic of clear-cell adenocarcinoma of the endometrium.

HSIL: immature squamous metaplastic-type cells, single or syncytia, enlarged hyperchromatic nuclei with contour irregularity, scant cytoplasm, high n:c; in liquid-based preparations the nuclei may appear less hyperchromatic.

Hyperchromatism: increase in the intensity of nuclear staining, i.e., increased basophilia.

Hyperkeratosis: thickening of the stratum corneum layer of epithelium.

Hyperplasia: increase in the number of cells.

Hypertrophy: increase in the size of tissue, by an increase in the size and the number of cells.

Immature squamous metaplasia: squamous metaplastic cells with high n:c.

Inclusions: contents of extraneous or abnormal intrinsic particles within the cytoplasm or the nucleus.

Inflammatory changes: reactive changes in the cytoplasm (e.g., altered staining) and the nucleus (e.g., blurred chromatin and prominent nucleoli).

Irradiation effect: cytomegaly, karyomegaly, vacuolation of cytoplasm and nucleus, polychromasia, etc.

Karyolysis: degenerative change; nucleus swells and loses chromatin.

Karyopyknotic index: one of the hormonal indices that indicates the percentage of cells with pyknotic nuclei among the intermediate and superficial cells. Highest karyopyknotic index is seen during ovulation.

Karyorrhexis: nuclear fragmentation.

Keratinization: orangeophilic staining of cytoplasm in keratinizing, dysplastic, and neoplastic squamous lesions on the Pap test.

Keratinizing dysplasia: keratinizing cells with nuclear and cytoplasmic atypia.

Koilocytes: enlarged superficial or intermediate cells, raisin-like nuclei, dense cytoplasm, empty, optically clear perinuclear cavity with sharp borders, manifestation of HPV-effect. *Koilos:* Greek for cavity.

Lactobacilli: also known as Doderlein's bacilli; thrive in low vaginal pH.

Leptothrix: filamentous microorganism that thrives with *Trichomonas vaginalis.*

LSIL: low-grade squamous intra-epithelial lesion; single cell or sheets of cells, nuclei are larger than three times the size of intermediate cell nuclei, hyperchromatic or smudged with membrane irregularities, relative increase in n:c ratio.

Lubricating jelly: may contaminate Pap smears; amorphous material with a blue tinge.

Lymphoglandular bodies: blue-staining cytoplasmic fragments in lymphoid lesions.

Maturation index: used to quantify the type of squamous cells. A minimum of 100 cells are counted, and the number of parabasal (P), intermediate (I), and superficial cells (S) are expressed as a ratio, i.e., P:I:S.

Menometrorrhagia: heavy or out-of-cycle vaginal bleeding of hormonal origin.

Metaplasia: transformation of one mature cell type to another mature cell type.

Microglandular hyperplasia: seen in the endocervix and is associated with oral contraceptives, hormone replacement therapy, and pregnancy; glandular pattern shows normal appearing endocervical cells with lumina formation; mimics adenocarcinoma, metaplastic pattern mimics ASC-H and HSIL; negative immunostaining with carcinoembryonic antigen.

"Moth-eaten" cells: appearance of squamous cells in trichomoniasis.

Multinucleated giant cells: could be epithelial, histiocytic, trophoblastic, or malignant.

Multiple nucleoli: seen in repair, high-grade carcinoma, glandular neoplasia.

Navicular cell: "boat-shaped cell;" variant of intermediate cell and is seen in pregnancy.

Necrosis: death of tissue characterized by nuclear changes.

Nucleolus: round-oval intranuclear eosinophilic structure with RNA.

Nucleus: membrane-lined intracytoplasmic body.

Orangeophilia: stains orange with OG-6 dye.

Parakeratotic cells: miniature superficial squamous cells.

"Pearl:" concentric structure with keratinized cells; nuclei are retained.

Pemphigus vulgaris: atypical squamous cells in sheets, high n:c, nuclei with smooth contour.

Perinuclear halo: vacuole around the nucleus; larger in HPV-infected cells; smaller in *Trichomonas* infection and in folic deficiency.

Phagocytosis: presence of particles or fragments within another cell.

Plasma cell: eccentric clock-face nucleus, dense cytoplasm, perinuclear clearing ("*hof*"), rarely seen in the Pap test; may indicate chronic endometritis, plasma cell cervicitis, or plasma cell dyscrasia.

Prominent nucleoli: seen in decidua, repair, squamous and glandular dysplasia and neoplasia.

Pseudokoilocytosis: perinuclear halo may be a result of glycogen content of the cell or inflammation.

Pseudoparakeratosis: glandular cells with orangeophilic cytoplasm seen with hormonal therapy; also known as the "pill effect."

Psammoma bodies: laminated calcifications in papillary ovarian tumors, endosalpingiosis, mesothelial hyperplasia, etc.

Puberty: replacement of atrophic vaginal mucosa in young girls by mature squamous cells that may show cyclic changes.

Pyknosis: nuclear shrinkage, condensation of chromatin to structureless mass.

Reactive endocervical cells: enlarged columnar cells with large round-to-oval nuclei, multinucleation with a single nucleolus, pale chromatin, and vacuolated cytoplasm.

Repair: sheets or syncytia of cells with a "streaming" effect; nuclei are enlarged with prominent nucleoli, chromatin remains even and finely granular, mitosis is seen, and inflammatory cells are present.

Regenerative changes: similar to repair; sheets or syncytia of cells with a "streaming" effect, nuclei are enlarged with prominent nucleoli, chromatin remains even and finely granular, mitosis is seen, and inflammatory cells are present.

Sheets: cell aggregates in a monolayer, regularly arranged.

Sperm in Pap smear: may be important in Pap smears from HIV-infected women, indicative of unprotected sexual relations.

Spindle cells: when present should rule out high-grade dysplasia, keratinizing squamous carcinoma, and sarcoma.

Squamous metaplasia: squamous cells with dense-to-delicate cytoplasm, smooth nuclear membranes with open chromatin, small nucleoli, and a "cobblestone" arrangement.

Syncytium: irregularly arranged cells with indistinct cell boundaries.

Therapy changes: cytomegaly and nucleomegaly, cells in sheets, pale nuclei with smooth contours, prominent nucleoli, nuclear and cytoplamic vacuoles, low n:c, mitoses, no single cells, polychromasia, and mimics nonkeratinizing squamous carcinoma.

Tingible-body macrophage: histiocytes with ingested nuclear debris from degenerating cells; seen in conditions of rapid cell turn over including follicular cervicitis, small-cell carcinoma, and malignant lymphoma.

Torulopsis glabrata: a form of *Candida* that may be symptomatic and difficult to distinguish from *Candida* on a Pap stain. No hyphal forms are seen in torulopsis.

Transformation zone: most SIL arise in the transformation zone—an area of variable size and extent wherein squamous metaplasia occurs. The T-zone recedes with age and may lie within the endocervical canal in older women.

Transitional cell metaplasia: can be seen in the uterine cervix and vagina, consists of several layers of small, uniform cells with intranulear grooves; may mimic HSIL.

Trichomonas vaginalis: ovoid protozoan, indistinct nucleus, cytoplasmic granules present; flagella may be seen on liquid-based preparations.

Trophoblastic cells: there are two types:

Syncytiotrophoblastic: 20+ nuclei, amphophilic cytoplasm, uniformly coarse irregular chromatin, nucleoli are rare.

Cytotrophoblastic: large cell, nucleus large and irregular, uniformly amphophilic cytoplasm, nucleus lobulated and may be vacuolated; difficult to distinguish from squamous cells.

Tubal metaplasia: metaplastic process of the endocervix with tubal-type ciliated epithelium more common in women aged 35 or older; also known as "ciliated cell" metaplasia, mimics glandular neoplasia particularly AIS.

Undifferentiated cells: cell lacking differentiation, organization, or specialization.

Vacuole: intracytoplasmic or intranuclear clear space with a sharp outline in intrauterine device use, radiation, glycogen, or glandular neoplasia.

Vaginal adenosis: glandular epithelium in the vagina, usually in dlethylstilbestrol exposure *in utero.*

Vesicular: uniformly delicate nuclear chromatin.

"Watery" diathesis: serous discharge, usually seen in endometrial carcinoma.

2

Analogies in the Pap Test

Of "Corn Flakes" and "Raisins"

Cytological Appearances of Cells in a Pap Smear Simulating Common Objects

Objects	Cytological counterpart
Ball-like	Endometrial carcinoma
Bamboo-like	*Geotrichium*
Bean-shaped	Nucleus of histiocyte
Blue balls	Menstrual endometrial cells; "exodus" refers to contour
Blue blobs	Degenerated parabasal cells in atrophic vaginits
Cannibalism	Ingested cytoplamic neutrophils in endometrial carcinoma
Cannonball	Aggregates of neutrophils in *Candida* and *Trichomonas*
Cartwheel	Nuclear chromatin in plasma cells
Cheesy	Discharge from *Candida* vaginitis
Clock-face	Nuclear chromatin in plasma cells
Clinging	Diathesis in squamous carcinoma on liquid-based preps
Clue cells	Bacilli covering intermediate cells—bacterial vaginosis
Cigar-shape	Nucleus of keratinizing squamous carcinoma
Cobblestone	Arrangement of squamous metaplastic cells
Cocklebur	Hematoidin crystals
Comet-like	Cytoplasm of low-grade endometrial sarcoma
Corkscrew	Churchman's spirals in endocervical mucus
Corn flakes	Trapped air under a cover slip; preparation artifact
Crushing	Nuclear DNA streaking in small-cell carcinoma
Daisy-like	Mesothelial hyperplasia in pelvic washings
Dirty	Background appearance of Pap test during menses
Dust ball	Appearance of *Actinomyces*
Exodus	Endometrial cells and stroma seen in days 7–10.
Feathering	Edges of endocervical adenocarcinoma *in situ*
Fenestrations	Glandular lumina in microglandular hyperplasia
Ferning	Estrogen effect on mucus
Fiber cells	Suggestive of invasive squamous cells
Fishy smell	Bacterial vaginosis; (+) "whiff" test
Flailing	Reparative endocervical cells pulled apart; cytoplasm from adjacent cells stretch out but remain attached
Ground-glass	Nuclei in herpesvirus infection

From: *Fundamentals of Pap Test Cytology*
By: R. S. Hoda and S. A. Hoda © Humana Press Inc., Totowa, NJ

Hair-like	Leptothrix (*Leptotrichia buccalis*)
Halo	Human papillomavirus (HPV) effect
Hand mirror	Trophoblastic cells
Histiocyte shower	Exodus during days 6–10 accompanied by endometrial cells
Hobnail	Cells in clear-cell type endometrial adenocarcinoma
Honeycomb	Endocervical cells viewed *en face*
Indian-filing	Linear array of metastatic lobular breast carcinoma
India-ink	Dark nuclei of keratinizing squamous-cell carcinoma
Kidney-shaped	Nucleus of histiocyte
Kite cells	HPV effect; refers to shape of cell
Koilocytes	Koilos = hollow or cavity in HPV
Leaf-like	Squamous metaplasia
Maltese-cross	Refractile starch contaminant
Mini cells	Cells of keratinized cells in parakeratosis
Molding	Nuclear arrangement in small-cell anaplastic carcinoma
Mosaic-like	Squamous metaplasia
Moth-eaten	Trichomoniasis-affected cells
Navicular	Boat-like (intermediate glycogenated) cells in pregnancy
Nuclear granules	Apoptotic bodies
Oat cell	Small-cell carcinoma of the cervix
Opaque	Degenerated nuclei in keratinizing squamous carcinoma
Pear	Refers to the shape of *Trichomonas vaginalis*
Pearl	Keratinized pearl of squamous cells
Peg cell	Nonsecretory cell higher up in the endocervical canal
Pencil cells	Elongated cells with tapered ends in an endocervical polyp
Permissive	Mature squamous cells that produce HPV virions
Picket-fence	Traumatically removed endocervical cells
Pill effect	Pseudoparakeratosis
Polka-dot	Keratohyaline granules in HPV
Pomegranate	Herpesvirus-molded nuclei
Porous	Cytoplasm in *Chlamydia trachomatis*
Raisin-like	Wrinkled nuclear membrane in HPV effect
Ratty	Background of cytolysis resulting from bacteria
Rosette	Cell groups in adenocarcinoma *in situ*
Salt and pepper	Nuclear chromatin in neuroendocrine tumors
Scavenger	Histiocytic cells with debris
School of fish	Arrangement of regenerative cells
Signet-ring	Intracellular mucin in metastatic lobular carcinoma
Small blue	Includes so-called tamoxifen-related cells
Smudge cells	Status-post laser, "smudging" appears in nucleus and cytoplasm
Snake-like	Elongated nuclei in atypical parakeratosis
Snowshoe	Alternaria, a contaminant
Soap bubble	Cytoplasmic vacuoles in radiation-therapy changes
Spaghetti and meatballs	*Candida*
Spider-like	Metaplastic cells pulled apart
Sticky cells	Superficial endometrial stromal cells
Strawberry	Colposcopic appearance of cervix: trichomonads

Streaming	Cells in repair
Sulfur granule	Seen in *Actinomyces*
Tadpole cells	Nuclei of invasive squamous carcinoma cells
Targetoid	Chlamydia inclusions
Tingible-body	Macrophages in follicular cervicitis; refers to phagocytized debris
Watery	Diathesis in endometrial carcinoma
Wrinkled cells	Progesterone effect in intermediate cells

3
Basic Cytology Principles

FEATURES TO BE EVALUATED IN A PAP TEST

- Adequacy.
- Presence of abnormal cells.
- Number and distribution of abnormal cells.
- Relationship between cells.
- Cell size and shape.
- Nuclear size and shape.
- Nuclear changes and nucleoli.
- Nuclear-to-cytoplasmic (n:c) ratio.
- Cytoplasmic features.
- Background or diathesis.

FEATURES OF PRENEOPLASTIC AND NEOPLASTIC CELLS

- Abnormality in size and shape of cells.
- Variation in cell size and shape.
- Increase in nuclear size.
- Increase in nuclear membrane irregularity.
- Hyperchromasia.
- Prominence of nucleoli and irregularity in shape thereof.
- Thickening of nuclear membrane.
- Increase in n:c ratio.
- Cytoplasm scanty.
- Mitosis, increased number, and abnormal forms.
- Noncohesiveness.
- Abnormal polarity.

COMMON CAUSES OF FALSE-NEGATIVE PAP TEST

- Atypical endocervical cells.
- Crowded cell aggregates.
- Cytolysis.
- Intermediate cells with nuclear enlargement.
- Keratinized cells.
- Metaplastic-like cells.
- Necrotic debris.
- Artifacts such as obscuring blood, inflammation, or air-drying.

From: *Fundamentals of Pap Test Cytology*
By: R. S. Hoda and S. A. Hoda © Humana Press Inc., Totowa, NJ

COMMON CAUSES OF FALSE-POSITIVE PAP TEST

- Atrophic smear.
- Atypical endocervical or endometrial cells.
- Multinucleated cells.
- Parakeratosis.
- Perinuclear halo in nonkoilocytes.
- Pseudoparakeratosis.
- Reactive/repair.
- Squamous metaplasia.
- Tubal metaplasia.

DIFFERENTIAL DIAGNOSIS OF CELLS WITH "NAKED" NUCLEI

- Autolysis of cytoplasm in menopause.
- Cytolysis.
- Degeneration, especially of endocervix.
- Reserve cells with tamoxifen treatment.

DIFFERENTIAL DIAGNOSIS OF GIANT MULTINUCLEATED CELLS

- Histiocytes.
- Atrophy.
- Folic acid deficiency.
- Tissue repair.
- Viral infection.
- Granuloma.
- Radiation.
- Syncytiotrophoblast.
- Squamous carcinoma.
- Choriocarcinoma.
- Uterine sarcoma.

CYTOLOGICAL FEATURES OF "DARK-CELL CLUSTERS"

- Crowded with piling up of cells.
- Hyperchromatic overlapping nuclei.
- Anisonucleosis.
- Scant cytoplasm.
- Increased n:c ratio.
- Mitosis present.
- Often difficult to determine whether squamous or glandular.

DIFFERENTIAL DIAGNOSIS OF "DARK-CELL CLUSTERS"

- Reactive endocervical cells.
- Tubal metaplasia.
- Atrophy: *nuclear membrane smooth*.
- Benign endometrial cells.

Table 1
Differential Diagnosis of "Small Blue" Cells in Pap Test

	Tamoxifen cells	Endometrial	Small-cell cancer	Breast cancer[a]
Architecture	Tight clusters	Tight clusters	Crowded sheets	Indian-files
Cells	Small, bland	Small, bland	Small, ovoid	Small, round
Nuclei	Dark, smooth	Irregular	Dark, irregular	Eccentric irregular
Nucleoli	(+/–)	(+), minute	(–)	(+)
Cytoplasm	Minimal	Minimal	Scanty	Vacuole
Necrosis	(–)	(–)	(+)	(–)
Mitoses	(–)	(–)	(+)	(–)

[a]Metastatic.

- Atypical squamous cells cannot exclude high-grade squamous intra-epithelial lesion.
- High-grade squamous intra-epithelial lesion: *nuclear membrane irregular.*
- Adenocarcinoma *in situ.*
- Endocervical or endometrial carcinoma.

DIFFERENTIAL DIAGNOSIS OF SMALL CELLS (TABLE 1)

- Lymphocytes in chronic lymphocytic cervicitis.
- Degenerated cells.
- Endometrial cells.
- Histiocytes.
- Reserve cells.
- Tamoxifen cells.
- Smaller cell type of squamous-cell carcinoma.
- Small-cell anaplastic carcinoma.

DIFFERENTIAL DIAGNOSIS OF CELLS WITH MACRONUCLEOLI

- Repair, regenerative, or reactive squamous cells.
- Reactive endocervical cells.
- Viral inclusions.
- Treatment effect.
- Decidua.
- Adenocarcinoma.
- Metastatic tumor.
- Nonkeratinizing squamous carcinoma.
- Pemphigus.

DIFFERENTIAL DIAGNOSIS OF ADENOCARCINOMA

- Viral infections.
- Endocervical cells, benign and atypical.

- Endometrial cells, benign and atypical.
- Endometritis.
- Histiocytes.
- Metaplasia.
- Vaginal adenosis.
- Intrauterine device.
- Microglandular hyperplasia.
- Metastatic tumor.

CLINICAL INFORMATION NEEDED
FOR OPTIMAL PAP TEST INTERPRETATION

- Patient's name.
- Age.
- Date of last menstrual period.
- Menopausal status.
- Presence of an intrauterine device.
- Pregnancy.
- Hormone treatment status.
- History of previous cytological abnormalities, cervical biopsies such as cone biopsies, or laser treatment.
- History of malignancy and subsequent chemotherapy and/or radiation therapy.

NOTA BENE

- Morphological expression of cell growth is best seen in the nucleus.
- Variation in cell size within a group of the same cell type is known as "anisonucleosis."
- Altered vaginal flora may result in multiple vaginal bacterial infection.

4

Basic Anatomy and Cytology
of the Female Genital Tract

INTRODUCTION

The female genital tract is composed of the vulva, vagina, uterus (cervix and body or corpus), fallopian tubes, and ovaries.

VULVA

The vulva consists of the mons pubis, labia majora, labia minora, clitoris, vestibule hymen, and Bartholin glands.

- *Mons pubis:* is a fat-filled prominence over the pubic bone. The mons and labia majora are covered by keratinized, stratified squamous epithelium with hair follicles, sebaceous glands, and sweat glands.
- *Labia majora and minora:* are anterior and posterior, respectively, and form the lateral borders of the vestibulum. The labia minora and prepuce are less keratinized and have sebaceous and sweat glands, as well as no hair follicles or underlying adipose tissue.
- *Vestibulum:* is the anterior space leading toward the vagina. It varies considerably in size and shape.
- *Hymen:* is a thin membrane that separates the vestibulum from the vagina in virgins.
- *Clitoris:* and the uretheral meatus are located above the vestibulum.

VAGINA

The vagina is a fibromuscular tube that extends from the vaginal opening to the cervix located posterior to the urinary bladder and anterior to the rectum. The normal adult vaginal mucosa has a wrinkled appearance.

The Bartholin glands are located posterior to the vestibulum, are tubulo-alveolar glands, and their excretory ducts are lined by transitional-type epithelium. They are located at either side of the vaginal opening. Bartholin's glands produce small amounts of lubricating fluid.

On **histology**, the vaginal wall consists of three layers—stratified nonkeratinizing squamous epithelium that rests on vascularized connective tissue with no glands or muscularis mucosae, and a layer of smooth muscle.

The **lymphatics** from the anterior and posterior portions of the vagina drain into the inguinal and pelvic lymph nodes, respectively.

From: *Fundamentals of Pap Test Cytology*
By: R. S. Hoda and S. A. Hoda © Humana Press Inc., Totowa, NJ

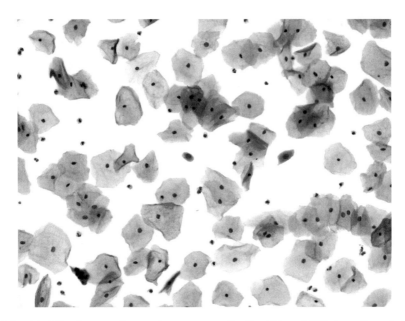

Fig. 4.1. Mixed types of normal squamous cells (liquid-based ThinPrep; Papanicolaou stain).

The squamous epithelium of the cervix and vagina is divided into three zones (*see* Figs. 4.1–4.5)

- *Basal layer:* composed of one or two layers of spherical cells resting on the basal lamina. Mitoses may be seen.
- *Intermediate layer:* thickest layer and is composed of cells that progressively mature toward the surface, nuclei are round with granular chromatin, and the cytoplasm is glycogenated.
- *Superficial layer:* consists of five to six layers of large flat eosinophilic cells with pyknotic nuclei (Tables 1 and 2).

CORPUS UTERUS

The corpus uterus is the main female internal reproductive organ. It consists of the body or the corpus, cervix, and endocervix. The uterine wall is composed of four layers—the inner epithelial layer consisting of a layer of cuboidal-to-columnar cells measuring 7–10 µm in length, a smooth muscle layer (myometrium), the serosa, and the peritoneum (covers only the body). The uterine cavity (endometrial cavity) is a triangular space, lined by the endometrium. The **endometrium** grows and changes during the menstrual cycle to prepare to receive a fertilized egg, and sheds a layer at the end of every menstrual cycle in the absence of fertilization. The endometrium undergoes various phases during the menstrual cycle, comprising the menstrual phase. The proliferative phase follows the menstrual phase and is under the influence of estrogens. It persists until ovulation (days 12–14). The secretory phase is postovulation and is under the influence of progesterone.

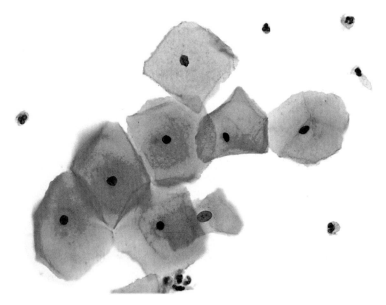

Fig. 4.2. Normal superficial cells are large and flat with pyknotic nuclei and eosinophilic cytoplasm (liquid-based ThinPrep; Papanicolaou stain).

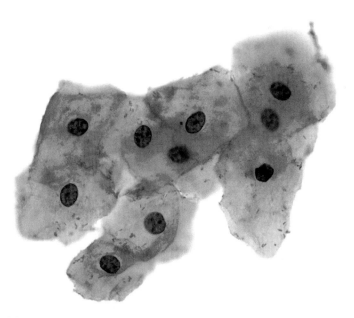

Fig. 4.3. Normal intermediate cells are large cells with small vesicular nuclei and cyanophilic or eosinophilic cytoplasm (liquid-based ThinPrep; Papanicolaou stain).

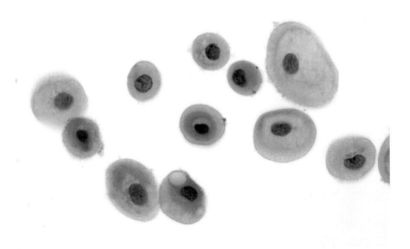

Fig. 4.4. Normal parabasal cells are usually singly dispersed, have a large uniform nucleus, and distinct cytoplasmic borders (liquid-based ThinPrep; Papanicolaou stain).

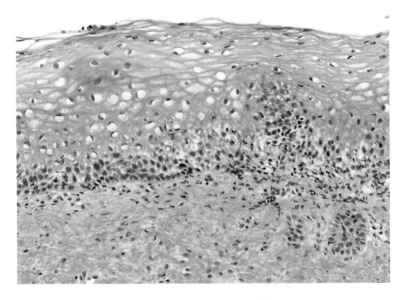

Fig. 4.5. Normal ectocervix (H&E stain).

Table 1
Squamous Cell Types in a Pap Smear (Figs. 4.2–4.4)

Features	Superficial cells	Intermediate cell	Parabasal cell
Cells	Singly	Singly	Singly
	Loose clustered	Loose clustered	Sheets
Shape	Polyhedral	Polyhedral, oval	Oval, round
Cell diameter	<25 µm,	~40 µm	~40 µm
Nucleus	<12 µm, pyknotic	<10 µm, vesicular	<6 µm, vesicular
	Fine chromatin	Fine chromatin	Fine chromatin
Cytoplasm	Transparent	Transparent	Opaque
	Granules	–	–
	Flat	Folded, flat	Flat

Table 2
Comparative Sizes of Cells Seen in Pap Smears (µm²)

Cell type	Cell area	Nuclear area
Superficial	1500	20
Intermediate	1500	35
Parabasal	300	50
Endocervical	200	50
Endometrial	175	30
Reserve cells	200	50

- *Cervix:* comprises of the lower third of the uterus and connects the uterus to the vagina via the endocervical canal. It has two parts: ectocervix and endocervix (Table 2).
- *Ectocervix:* lined by nonkeratinizing, stratified squamous epithelium similar to the vaginal mucosa and shows maturation from the basal layer to the surface.
- *Endocervix:* lined by of single layer of tall, columnar mucus-secreting cells with round-to-oval basally located nuclei with vesicular chromatin. These cells also line the endocervical glands present in the cervical stroma. Nabothian cysts form when the openings of these glands are plugged by mucus. The cells in the upper portion of the endocervical canal may be ciliated (tubal metaplasia).
- *Squamocolumnar junction:* also known as the transformation zone (TZ) is the point where the stratified squamous epithelium of the ectocervix meets the endocervical glandular epithelium. The position of the TZ varies with age.

In adolescents and young adults (and in certain pathological conditions), the endocervical epithelium is seen on the surface of the ectocervix (ectropion). Ectropion appears as red patches on colposcopy. During the reproductive years, the TZ is closer to the external os and during menopause it recedes into the endocervical canal. This zone is the site of origin for squamous intra-epithelial lesion and squamous carcinoma.

The **internal os**, or the isthmus, is the point of transition between the endometrial cavity and the endocervical canal. The **external os** is the opening of the endocervical canal into the vagina. The cervical os is mostly small and round in nulliparous women. It becomes slit-like (fish-mouth shape) after one or more pregnancies.

FALLOPIAN TUBES

Also known as oviducts, the fallopian tubes extend from the cornua of the endometrial cavity to the peritoneal cavity where it has a fimbriated end. It measures 7–14 cm in length, and 5–8 mm in circumference. The tube has four layers—the mucosa consisting of ciliated epithelium, a muscular layer, serosa, and peritoneum. After ovulation, the ovum travels via the fallopian tube, a process that takes days, to reach the uterus, propelled by the ciliated epithelium of the fallopian tube.

OVARIES

The ovaries are oval in shape and measure 4 cm in greatest dimension. The external surface of the ovary is smooth until puberty, whence it becomes irregular and lobulated as a result of scars from rupture of ovarian follicles. The ovaries perform two functions: the production of estrogen and progesterone, the female sex hormones, and the production of mature ova, or eggs. At birth, the ovaries contain nearly 400,000 ova, far more than the woman will need, because during an average reproductive lifespan the woman undergoes approx 500 menstrual cycles. After maturing, the egg travels down the fallopian tube, which takes 3 or 4 days. If the ovum becomes fertilized, it is embedded into the endometrium. Eggs that are not fertilized are expelled during menstruation.

NORMAL VAGINAL FLORA

Lactobacilli (Fig. 4.6)

- Also known as bacillus of Doderlein, *lactobacilli* are Gram-positive, unencapsulated, rod-shaped organisms that are part of the normal microbiological flora of the vagina.
- Maintain the normal pH of the vagina (3.9–4.2) by converting glycogen to lactic acid, thus preventing pathogenic bacterial growth.
- This enzymatic process is cytologically characterized as cytolysis and results in the destruction of the cytoplasm of intermediate cells.
- A Pap test shows numerous rods causing lysis of the cytoplasm, resulting in "bare" nuclei devoid of cytoplasm.
- Marked cytolysis may be seen in conditions where intermediate cells predominate, such as pregnancy and the secretory phase of menstrual cycle.
- Neutrophils may not be seen in large numbers.
- In women without bacterial vaginosis, the *lactobacillus* species is the most common bacteria (83 to 100% of clones).

SQUAMOUS METAPLASIA (FIGS. 4.7 AND 4.8)

- Is the conversion of columnar epithelium of the endocervix at the TZ to stratified squamous epithelium.

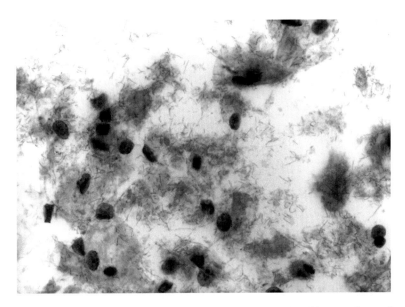

Fig. 4.6. Cytolysis with numerous *lactobacilli* causing the lysis of intermediate cell cytoplasm (liquid-based ThinPrep; Papanicolaou stain).

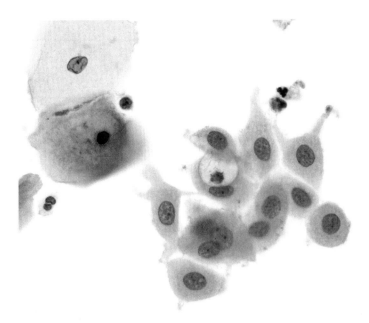

Fig. 4.7. Squamous metaplasia shows uniform, pale nuclei with small nucleoli and vacuolated cytoplasm. Cytoplasmic processes are seen when the cells are forcibly removed during sampling (liquid-based ThinPrep; Papanicolaou stain).

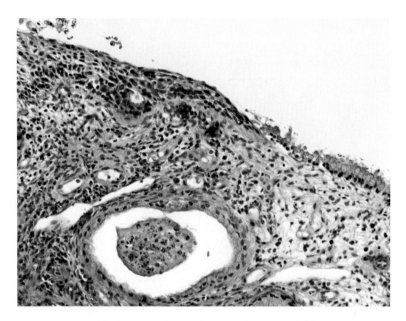

Fig. 4.8. Squamocolumnar junctional mucosa (H&E stain).

Table 3
Squamous Metaplasia vs SIL

	Squamous metaplasia	SIL
Cells	Flattened	Isolated
Nucleus	Small	Larger
	<Nucleus of intermed cell	>Nucleus of intermed cell
	Fine chromatin	Coarse chromatin
	Contour: smooth	Contour: wrinkled, wavy
Cytoplasm	More	Less

SIL, squamous intraepithelial lesion.

- It is a physiological phenomenon that may begin at puberty and continues throughout the reproductive years and beyond.
- May be related either to hormonal alterations or reactive changes to irritation or inflammation (Table 3).
- Thought to originate from reserve cells located just beneath the columnar endocervical-type epithelium.
- Cells are similar in appearance to parabasal cells.
- Nuclei are round and smooth with fine chromatin and small nucleoli.
- Cytoplasm is dense or may show vacuolations.
- Cytoplasmic projections that look like "spider legs" may be seen as a result of sampling.
- Presence of squamous metaplastic cells indicate that the TZ has been sampled.

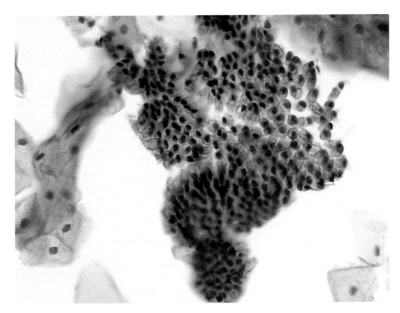

Fig. 4.9. Normal endocervical cells seen en face as a sheet with a honeycomb pattern (liquid-based SurePath; Papanicolaou stain).

ENDOCERVICAL CELLS (FIGS. 4.9 AND 4.10)

- Columnar cells with basally located nuclei.
- Cyanophilic cytoplasm that may be vacuolated.
- When seen from above, the cells are in a honeycomb sheet.
- When viewed on side the cells have a "picket-fence" arrangement.
- Chromatin is fine with small nucleoli.

ENDOMETRIAL CELLS (FIGS. 4.11 AND 4.12)

- Cytological appearance of endometrial cells vary with the phase of the menstrual cycle and the level of preservation.
- In a well-preserved state, the epithelial cells occur in tight three-dimensional cluster.
- Nuclei are small, round, and dark.
- Nucleoli are not usually seen.
- Cytoplasm is scant and may show vacuoles.
- Superficial stromal cells are round, histiocytic type, and stick together.
- Deep stromal cells are spindled and dark.
- Exodus is seen from day 6 to 10 of the menstrual cycle and consists of a central core of stromal cells surrounded by epithelial cells. Immunocytochemical analysis can be performed using CD10 for stromal and cytokeratin for epithelial cells, if needed.

RESERVE CELLS

- Totipotent cells seen at a subcolumnar location.
- Cells are small, round, and overlapping.

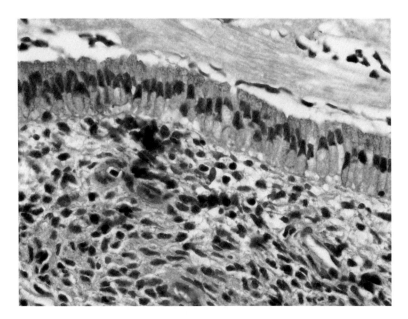

Fig. 4.10. Normal endocervix (H&E stain).

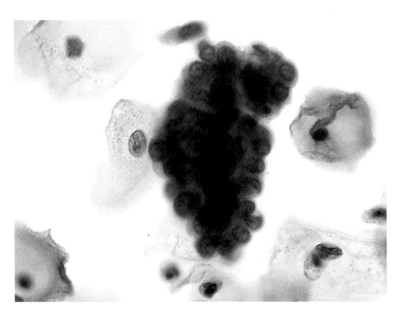

Fig. 4.11. Normal endometrial epithelial cells in a small cluster with scalloped borders, small cells with small nuclei, and occasional cytoplasmic vacuoles (liquid-based SurePath; Papanicolaou stain).

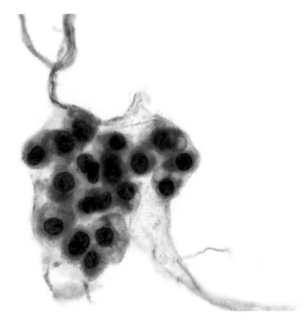

Fig. 4.12. Normal endometrial stromal cells, also known as "sticky" cells are seen as a small group with regular pale nuclei and delicate cytoplasm (liquid-based ThinPrep; Papanicolaou stain).

- Nuclei are small, dark, and uniform.
- Cytoplasm is either extremely scant or absent.
- Reserve cells may be seen with tamoxifen treatment.
- Reserve cells may give rise to small-cell neuroendocrine carcinoma of the cervix.
- May mimic endometrial cells.

5

The Bethesda System

Specimen Type: Conventional Smear (Pap Smear) vs Liquid-Based Preparations vs Other

Specimen adequacy
  Satisfactory for evaluation
  Unsatisfactory for evaluation
General categorization (optional)
  Negative for intra-epithelial lesion or malignancy
  Epithelial cell abnormality
  Other: *see* interpretation/result
  (e.g., endometrial cells in a woman ≥40 years)
Automated review
Ancilliary testing
Interpretation/result
  Negative for intra-epithelial lesion or malignancy
  Other
  Epithelial cell abnormalities
    Squamous cell
      Atypical squamous cells
        Of undetermined significance
        Cannot exclude high-grade squamous intra-epithelial lesion (HSIL)
      Low-grade squamous intra-epithelial lesion HSIL
      Squamous-cell carcinoma
    Glandular cell
      Atypical
        Endocervical cells (not otherwise specified [NOS] or specify in comments)
        Endometrial cells (NOS or specify in comments)
        Glandular cells (NOS or specify in comments)
      Atypical
        Endocervical cells, favor neoplastic
        Glandular cells, favor neoplastic
        Endocervical adenocarcinoma *in situ*
      Adenocarcinoma
        Endocervical
        Endometrial
        Extrauterine
        NOS
Other malignant neoplasms: (*specify*)
Educational notes and suggestions (*optional*)

From: *Fundamentals of Pap Test Cytology*
By: R. S. Hoda and S. A. Hoda © Humana Press Inc., Totowa, NJ

SPECIMEN ADEQUACY

Satisfactory for Evaluation

Minimum number of squamous cells in an adequate Pap smear test:

- *Conventional:* 8000–12,000, well-preserved, well-visualized.
- *Liquid-based:* ≥5000, well-preserved, well-visualized.

Unsatisfactory for Evaluation

- *Specimen rejected/not processed (specify reason):* including unlabeled specimen vial or slide, broken slide.
- *Specimen processed and examined, but unsatisfactory for evaluation of epithelial abnormality because of (specify reason):* including a scant ectocervical component, blood, inflammation (or other elements); obscure greater than 75% of the epithelial cells.
  - Note the presence of organisms or benign endometrial cells.

Determination of Adequacy Criteria for Conventional Pap Smears

- Conventional Pap smears are evaluated at ×4 magnification for a sufficient number of fields.
  - *Satisfactory:*
- If a ×4 field has 1000 cells, the specimen should have at least eight such ×4 fields to be adequate.
- If a ×4 field has 1400 cells, the specimen should have at least six such ×4 fields to be adequate.
  - *Unsatisfactory:*
- Less than 150 cells at ×4 objective in all microscopic fields.

Minimum Adequacy Criteria for Liquid-Based Preparations

- An adequate liquid-based preparation should have a greater than or equal to 5000 well visualized and preserved squamous cells.
- Ten microscopic fields are counted at ×10 or ×40 magnification starting at the edge of the specimen along any diameter (horizontal or vertical) that includes the center of the preparation.
- Hypocellular areas and "holes" in the preparation are included in proportion to their size.
- **ThinPrep:** has a 20-mm diameter circle. At ×10 and ×40 objective and an ocular with field number (FN) 20, there should be 50.0 and 3.1 cells, respectively, and at ×10 and ×40 objective and an ocular with FN22, there should be 60.5 and 3.8 cells, respectively.
- **SurePath:** has a 13-mm diameter circle. At ×10 and ×40 objective and an ocular with FN20, there should be 118.3 and 7.4 cells, respectively, and at ×10 and ×40 objective and an ocular with FN22, there should be 143.2 and 9.0 cells, respectively.

Quantitative Parameters of Partially Obscured and Unsatisfactory Paps

- *Satisfactory but partially obscured:* 50–75% of epithelial cells are obscured.
- *Unsatisfactory:* more than 75% of epithelial cells are obscured.
- *Note:* any specimen with epithelial abnormality is satisfactory for evaluation regardless of cellularity.

Determination of Representation of Transformation Zone

- At least 10 well-preserved endocervical or squamous metaplastic cells, not necessarily in clusters.

GENERAL CATEGORIZATION (OPTIONAL)

- Negative for intra-epithelial lesion or malignancy.
- Other: includes endometrial cells in a woman 40 years of age or older.
- Epithelial cell abnormality.

AUTOMATED REVIEW

If the case is examined by an automated device, indicate whether the scanning was successful, the device, and the manufacturer's name.

ANCILLARY TESTING

Include the method (name and brief description) used for reflex human papillomavirus (HPV) test, such as hybrid capture II, polymerase chain reaction, or *in situ* hybridization.

Results for reflex HPV test can be reported as:

- A result only.
- As a result with a recommendation for clinical management.
- As a result plus the probability of an associated dysplasia.
- As a definitive interpretation.

INTERPRETATION/RESULT

Negative for Intra-Epithelial Lesion or Malignancy

When there is no cellular evidence of neoplasia, state this in the General Categorization previously mentioned and/or in the Interpretation/Result section of the report, indicate whether or not there are organisms or other nonneoplastic findings.

Organisms

- *Trichomonas vaginalis.*
- Fungal organisms morphologically consistent with *Candida* spp.
- Shift in flora suggestive of bacterial vaginosis.
- Bacteria morphologically consistent with *Actinomyces* spp.
- Cellular changes consistent with herpes simplex virus.

Other Non-Neoplastic Findings (Optional to Report; List Not Inclusive)

Reactive cellular changes associated with:

- Inflammation (includes typical repair).
- Radiation.
- Intrauterine contraceptive device.
- Glandular cells status post-hysterectomy.
- Atrophy.

Other

- Endometrial cells (in a woman ≥40 years of age).
- Note that no squamous intra-epithelial lesion is identified (*see* Chapter 13).

Epithelial Cell Abnormalities

Squamous Cell

- Atypical squamous cells of undetermined significance.
- Atypical squamous cells cannot exclude high-grade squamous intra-epithelial lesion.
- Low-grade squamous intra-epithelial lesion, encompasses HPV/mild dysplasia/ cervical intra-epithelia neoplasia (CIN) 1.
- High-grade squamous intra-epithelial lesion, encompasses moderate-to-severe dysplasia, CIN 2,CIN 3/carcinoma *in situ*.
- Suspicious for invasive squamous-cell carcinoma.
- Squamous-cell carcinoma.

Glandular Cell

- Atypical.
  - Glandular cells, NOS.
  - Endocervical cells.
  - Endometrial cells, NOS.
- Atypical.
  - Endocervical cells, favor neoplastic.
  - Glandular cells, favor neoplastic.
- Endocervical adenocarcinoma *in situ*.
- Adenocarcinoma.
  - Endocervical.
  - Endometrial.
  - Extrauterine.
  - NOS.

Other Malignant Neoplasms

- Includes sarcoma, malignant lymphoma, and others.

EDUCATIONAL NOTES AND SUGGESTIONS

Suggestions are optional, and should be carefully crafted, concise, and consistent with published clinical follow-up guidelines (*see* Chapter 19).

6

Liquid-Based Preparations

INTRODUCTION

The liquid-based cytology sample preparations (liquid-based preparation [LBP]) include ThinPrep (TP) (Cytyc Corp, Marlborough, MA) and SurePath (SP) (TriPath Imaging Inc., Burlington, NC). In both of these systems, instead of smearing cells on a slide, cells are rinsed into a liquid collection media containing fixatives. This ensures the capture of an entire sample from the collection devices. For conventional smears, most of the sample (~80%) is discarded with the sampling device. Despite the difference in preparatory techniques, the two LBP, TP and SP, are similar in appearance (Table 1).

ADVANTAGES OF LBP

- Almost 100% of the collected cells are captured, processed, and reviewed.
- Immediate liquid fixation prevents artifacts, such as air-drying.
- Easier to review slides (Tables 2 and 3).
- Smaller screening area (TP, 20-mm and SP, 13-mm).
- Preparatory technique reduces debris, cell clumps and obscuring elements.
- Cleaner background.
- Significantly fewer unsatisfactory cases.
- Homogenized specimen.
- Increased detection of high-grade squamous intra-epithelial lesions and above.
- Ancillary testing such as reflex human papillomavirus (HPV) test and other molecular tests (Chlamydia/gonorrhea), immunocytochemistry can be performed from the residual material.
- Potential for processing residual material as a cell block.

PREPARATION OF LBP SPECIMENS

TP Preparation Technique

1. Specimen collection and fixation. Sample is collected using either a broom-type device or a plastic spatula and endocervical brush combination. The collection device is then rinsed in a specimen vial containing PreservCyt solution, a methanol-based fixative, which also lyses blood.
   Specimen is labeled and transported to the cytology laboratory.
2. Steps in preparation. TP processor is a semi-automated device and comes in two versions. TP2000 processes one specimen at a time. TP3000 batch processes 80 specimens at one time. The microscopic slides used for the ThinPrep Pap Test are provided by Cytyc Corp and are marked with a 20-mm diameter circle. The specimen vial and the

From: *Fundamentals of Pap Test Cytology*
By: R. S. Hoda and S. A. Hoda © Humana Press Inc., Totowa, NJ

Table 1
Appearances on Liquid-Based Preparations

- **Adenocarcinoma** *in situ*, **endocervix:** nuclei show "feathering" and stippled chromatin.
- **Atypical squamous cells cannot exclude high-grade squamous intra-epithelial lesion:** cells may be smaller.
- **Atypical squamous cells of undetermined significance (ASC-US):** features of ASC-US are easily appreciated because of better cell preservation.
- **Atrophy:** nuclei appear smaller, autolysis ("bare" nuclei) is less common, pseudoparakeratotic cells may appear orangeophilic, and granular background debris is clumped and is similar to the granular diathesis of squamous-cell carcinoma. The distinction is made by the absence of malignant squamous cells in atrophy.
- *Candida* **spp.:** organisms stain eosinophilic to gray-brown. There is "spearing" of squamous cells along the long axis of organisms.
- **Coccobacilli:** cells are covered with *coccobacilli* and background is cleaner.
- **Endometrial cells:** cells tend to round up in three-dimensional clusters, intracytoplasmic vacuoles are more evident, and small nucleoli are visible in normal cells.
- **Follicular cervicitis:** lymphoid cells may appear in clusters and may mimic endometrial cells.
- **Repair:** less "streaming;" groups may appear more rounded, frayed cytoplasmic edges may be seen, and staining may be uniform with less polychromasia.
- *Trichomonas vaginalis:* Organisms appear smaller, eosinophilic granules are better seen, and flagella are preserved.

Additional morphology described in other chapters.

labeled slide are placed into the TP processor. Preparatory steps include specimen dispersion, collection, and transfer.

    a. Dispersion. A disposable cylinder with a polycarbonate filter attached to one end is introduced into the vial. The pore size of the filter is 8 µm (pore size for nongynecological specimens is 5.5 µm). The instrument disaggregates blood, mucus, debris, and breaks up large cell clusters, mixes and homogenizes the cell suspension by spinning, either the cylinder (TP2000) or the vial (TP3000), for a few seconds.

    b. Collection. A gentle vacuum is applied to the cylinder that aspirates the cell suspension through the filter. Most of the broken red blood cells and debris is allowed to pass through while the diagnostic cells attach and remain on the external surface of the filter. The instrument monitors cell density across the filter and the flow rate decreases when cells are evenly distributed on the filter with minimal cell overlap.

    c. Transfer. The cylinder moves out of the specimen, is inverted 180°, is gently pressed against a positively charged slide, and with slight positive pressure, transfers the cells (~70,000) to the glass slide. The slide is immediately dropped into 95% ethanol fixative. Preparation time ranges between 30 and 90 seconds depending on cell concentration. Papanicolaou staining is either performed manually or in an automatic stainer. The staining process takes 30 minutes.

3. Residual specimen. The shelf life of the residual specimen is 3 months at room temperature. It can be used for reflex HPV test, other molecular tests, such as those for chlamydia and gonorrhea, and immmunocytochemistry. TP has been approved by the FDA for the aforementioned molecular tests. TP can also be used to process multiple representative slides or a cell block.

Table 2
General Cytological Features on Liquid-Based Preparations
and Conventional Smear

Features	ThinPrep	SurePath	Conventional smear
Background			
Clean	Yes	Yes	No
RBCs	Reduced	Reduced	Present/usually obscures
Neutrophils	Reduced	Reduced	Present/usually obscures
Necrosis	Clumped	Clumped	Diffuse/usually obscures
Cellularity	Adequate	Adequate	Adequate
Cell preservation	Good	Good	+/–
Cell distribution	Uniform	Uniform to uneven	Uniform to uneven
	One plane	Different planes	–
Cell size	Smaller	Smaller	Larger
Architecture	Preserved	Preserved	Preserved
Cytomorphology	Preserved	Preserved	Preserved
EC material			
Quantity	Reduced	Reduced	–
Quality	Clumped	Clumped	Diffuse
Artifacts	None	None	Usually +[a]
Slide evaluation	Easier	Easy to difficult	Easy to difficult
Reproducibility	(+)	(+)	Usually not
Ancillary studies	Possible	Possible	Usually not

[a]Air-drying thick and obscured cell groups.
RBCs, red blood cells; EC, extracellular.

Table 3
Specific Cellular Features of Liquid-Based Preparations
and Conventional Smears

Features	ThinPrep	SurePath	Conventional
Cellular overlap	Minimal	Increased	Increased
Architectural distortion	+	+	+
Fragmentation	+	+	–
Monolayer cells	+	–	N/A
Sheets of cells	+, small	+, small	larger
Cell clusters	+, thin	++, thick, 3D	++
Cellular elongation	–	+	–
Nuclear detail	Good	Good	Good
Membrane irregularity	+	+	+
Chromatin detail	Preserved	Preserved	Preserved
Nucleoli	Preserved	Preserved	Preserved
Cytoplasm detail	Good	Good	Good

SP Preparation Technique

1. Specimen collection and fixation. Sample is collected using a broom-type device or a combination of the endocervical brush/plastic spatula. The tip of the collection device is detached into a specimen vial containing a proprietary solution (CytoRich), which is an ethanol-based fixative. Detaching the device heads into the vial ensures capturing the entire specimen. The specimen is labeled and transported to the cytology laboratory.
2. Steps in specimen preparation
   a. Vortexing. A multi-vortexor mixes 25 samples at a time.
   b. Loading the specimens in the PrepMate. The PrepMate instrument continues the homogenization process using a syringing technique and it also then layers 8–10 cc of the sample over the density gradient in a centrifuge tube. Twelve samples are processed on the PrepMate in 3 minutes.
   c. Cell enrichment process. The sample is centrifuged in a Hettich centrifuge twice to pull the cell solution through the density gradient. The density gradient is formulated to fractionate cells from obscuring artifacts such as blood, mucus, inflammation, and protein using size, weight, and density. In essence the cells are concentrated. The cell pellet is considered enriched because it contains primarily epithelial cells. The first centrifuge is at $200g$ for 2 minutes. The supernatant is decanted and the specimen is centrifuged again at $800g$ for 10 minutes and decanted. Both steps are done using a batch method of processing 48 samples at one time.
   d. PrepStain Slide Processor. The enriched cell samples which are in centrifuge tubes are placed on the PrepStain slide processor where the cell pellet is re-suspended automatically by the instrument.
   e. Cell-to-slide transfer. A robotic arm in the PrepStain transfers the sample from the tubes to a settling chamber that sits atop the glass slides. Cells are allowed to settle on the slides by gravity. The PrepStain can either stain each slide with the Pap stain, or slides can be taken off and stained according to standard laboratory protocol. This is called Prep Only. For PrepStain, approx 48 slides can be processed in 1 hour. For Prep only approx 96 slides can be processed in 1 hour (unstained).

The SP slides are freshly prepared in the laboratory for daily use. The slides are coated with a modified poly-L-lysine and air-dried. These positively charged slides allow diagnostic cells to settle out of solution and adhere to the surface. On completion, a thin layer of cells (~75,000) are deposited in a 13-mm diameter circle. Preparation time is usually 60 minutes for 48 stained slides. The shelf life of the residual material is 4 weeks at room temperature and 6 months at 4°C (refrigerated). SP is not FDA approved for reflex HPV test. However, laboratories use it (off-label) after validation studies. Residual material can be used to process multiple representative slides or a cell block.

AUTOMATION OF PAP TEST SCREENING

Currently, there are two automated slide scanning system, TP Imaging System (Cytyc Corp., Marlborough, MA) and FocalPoint Slide Profiler (TriPath Inc, Burlington, NC).

The TP Imaging System

The TP Imaging System is an automated imaging and review system indicated for primary screening of Pap tests. The system consists of three components, an image processor, a PC-based computer that runs on Windows NT (Microsoft Corp., Redmond, WA), and a review microscope with a mechanical stage and electronic dotting capability. The system can image more than 300 slides per day and holds 10 cartridges of 25 slides each. Once a cassette is imaged it is replaced by another one for continued imaging. The slides are barcoded for patient identification. The computer is designed to capture and analyze slide images and store the results of slide analyses after imaging. In a TP slide the cells are deposited in a 20-mm diameter circle. Normally, it would take 120 fields of vision (FOV) to screen the entire slide. The computer-based image processor scans the entire microscope slide and selects only 22 FOV (25% of the slide) with the most abnormal cells for review and stores the x- and y-coordinates of these cells in the computer. At the review scope, the barcode of the imaged slide is scanned and the manual stage will automatically allow the cytotechnologist to examine the 22 selected FOV. The automated stage has programmable screening preferences so that the cytotechnologist can set the screening direction and speed. A Pod is used to control the microscope. An automated marker allows the cytotechnologist to mark cells of interest for further review. The area of interest is marked by an "L." If a slide is marked, the cytotechnologist then manually reviews the entire slide. If an abnormality is detected, the slide is reviewed by a cytopathologist. Slides scanned by the imaging system are stained by a proprietary stain called the TP Stain, which emphasizes the nuclei. This stain is very similar to the traditional Pap stain.

Advantages of TP Imaging System

- Small size of the system.
- Motorized microscope stage prevents wrist injuries in cytotechnologists.
- Fewer fields of vision to review.
- Standardized Pap stain.

Limitations of TP Imaging System

- Not compatible with the traditional Pap staining method.
- Not compatible with conventional Pap smear slides.

FocalPoint Slide Profiler

The FocalPoint Slide Profiler is a fully automated instrument that classifies Pap test slides without human intervention. The instrument is FDA approved for primary screening of SP and conventional Pap smears.

The instrument can hold 36 trays of eight slides each and can thus process 288 slides per day. The device uses algorithms to measure nuclear features such as size, optical density, membrane, and nuclear-to-cytoplasmic ratio. The slides are barcoded and loaded onto trays. The system detects morphological changes associated with abnormal cells and specimen adequacy, and ranks the slides according to their likelihood of being abnormal. Up to 25% of the slides can be archived for no further review. Of the remaining 75% of the slides that require further review, at least 15% are identified for quality control rescreening.

Advantages of FocalPoint Slide Profiler
- Compatible with both SP and conventional Pap smears.
- Reduces the number of slides for actual screening.

Limitations of FocalPoint Slide Profiler
- Not compatible with all staining techniques.
- Performance characteristics for reactive changes, atrophy, 40 or more endometrial cells, and unusual tumors have not been established.
- Not approved for use in a high-risk patient population.
- All the slides selected for review have to be manually screened.

FIXATION OF THE PAP SMEAR

The specimen should be fixed immediately after procurement for optimal cell preservation. Conventional smears can be fixed in 95% ethyl alcohol for 15 minutes and then allowed to dry, or they can also be spray-fixed. Spray fixatives contain isopropanol and polyethylene glycol (carbowax) that protects the cells from drying. The nozzle of the spray fixative should be about 12-inches away from the surface of the slide for optimal fixation of cells. The slides are then transported to the laboratory in cardboard containers. The carbowax should be removed by washing smears in 50% alcohol for 5–10 minutes before staining them.

LBP are fixed immediately upon collection in the fixative sample collection media.

Papanicolaou Stain
- Papanicolaou stain the universal stain used for staining Pap test slides.
- Hematoxylin (Harris') is the nuclear stain. The blue color of the nucleus is enhanced by alum.
- Orange-G, eosin alcohol, lighter green, and bismarck brown are the cytoplasmic stains.

DETERMINATION OF ADEQUACY ON LBP

Please *see* Chapter 5.

7

Physiological Cytology

INTRODUCTION

Any physiological changes in a Pap test, without cellular changes of preneoplasia or neoplasia, are mentioned under the interpretation/result category of "negative for intra-epithelial lesion or malignancy."

Physiological Effects
Hormonal effects
Atrophy
Pregnancy

HORMONAL EVALUATION

- Used in evaluating the hormonal status for monitoring pregnancy, determining timing of ovulation for fertility workup, and artificial insemination.
- Vaginal smear allows rapid evaluation of ovarian function in women with disorders of menstruation.
- Smear should be taken by gentle scraping of the upper third of the lateral vaginal wall.
- Smear should be devoid of organisms, inflammation, and glandular cells.
- Patient should not be on hormone therapy or status postsurgery.
- Sequential smears are obtained to assess variability in pattern.
- Clinical information, such as age and last menstrual period, should be obtained.
- Although a variety of maturation indices are available, the most commonly utilized index is the maturation index (MI).
- MI is used to quantify the type of squamous cells.
- A minimum of 100 cells are counted and the number of parabasal (P), intermediate (I), and superficial (S) cells are expressed as a ratio (P:I:S). For example, the MI of a smear taken during the latter part of the postpartum period is expressed as 30:40:30, indicating mild maturation.

HORMONAL EFFECTS SEEN ON PAP TEST

Phases	P:I:S
• Birth	0:95:0
• Infancy—early childhood	100:0:0
• Late childhood	10:90:0
• Premenarche	0:70:30

From: *Fundamentals of Pap Test Cytology*
By: R. S. Hoda and S. A. Hoda © Humana Press Inc., Totowa, NJ

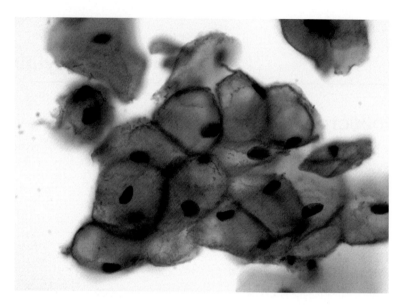

Fig. 7.1. Pregnancy, navicular cells (ThinPrep; Papanicolaou stain).

- Reproductive period
    - Preovulation   0:20:80
    - Ovulation   0:40:60
    - Postovulation   0:80:20
    - Pregnancy   0:95:5
    - Birth control pill   0:95:5
    - Threatened abortion   0:90:10
    - Spontaneous abortion   0:80:20
    - Postpartum, immediate   100:0:0
    - Postpartum, later   30:40:30
- Atrophy   70:30:0 or 30:70:0

Predominant Cell Types at Various Ages

Age	Predominant cell type
Neonate	Intermediate (effect of maternal hormones)
Prepubertal	Atrophic
Pubertal	Superficial
Menstrual	Intermediate, superficial plus blood
Preovulation	Superficial
Postovulation	Intermediate
Pregnancy (Fig. 7.1)	Intermediate, navicular (distinguish from koilocyte; Fig. 7.2)
Postpartum (Fig. 7.3)	Parabasal
Lactation	Parabasal
Postmenopause	Intermediate or parabasal or basal

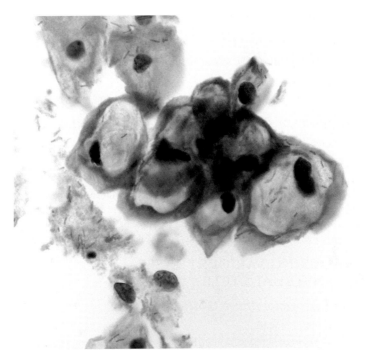

Fig. 7.2. Koilocytes. Note perinuclear halo (ThinPrep; Papanicolaou stain).

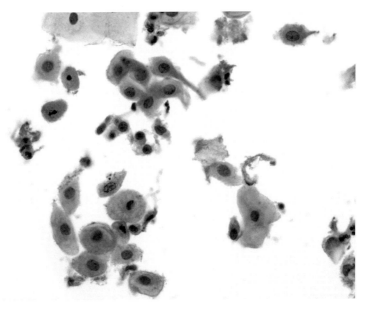

Fig. 7.3. Postpartum changes, parabasal cells (ThinPrep; Papanicolaou stain).

PHYSIOLOGICAL CHANGES

Hormonal Effects of Estrogen on Vaginal Epithelium

Effect does not depend on the smear pattern prior to therapy.

- Produces a very high maturation effect.
- Pregnancy is the only condition when women do not respond to hormones.

Hormonal Effects of Progesterone on Vaginal Epithelium

Effects depend on the status of the smear prior to therapy.

- In smears with high maturation there is regression to a less mature pattern with intermediate cells.
- In an atrophic smear, some degree of maturation occurs with an intermediate cell pattern.
- During pregnancy or the second half of the menstrual cycle, there is no change in the cell pattern, with persistence of the intermediate cell pattern.
- Arias–Stella-like changes occur in endocervical cells with long-term progesterone use.

PAP TEST DURING VARIOUS PHASES OF THE MENSTRUAL CYCLE

Pap Test in Estrogenic Phase (Follicular Phase)

- Superficial cells dominate.
- The cells occur singly and flat, with pyknotic nuclei and eosinophilic cytoplasm.
- Clean background with minimal inflammatory cells.
- Endocervical cells have a basophilic cytoplasm with centrally placed round nuclei.

Pap Test at Ovulation

- Superficial cells.
- Endocervical cells are swollen and large; nuclei show nipple-like protrusions.
- Cytoplasm is abundant and vacuolated.

Pap Test During Progestational Phase (Luteal Phase)

- Superficial cells are replaced by intermediate cells.
- Intermediate cells have folded cytoplasm and occur in sheets and clusters.
- Cytolysis present with many "bare" nuclei.
- Increased number of leukocytes.
- Dirty background.

PHYSIOLOGICAL AND PATHOLOGICAL CHANGES IN HORMONAL PATTERN

Atrophic Smear Pattern (Tables 1–4)

- Infancy and childhood.
- Postpartum and lactation.
- Menopause.
- Ovarian dysgenesis.
- Turner's syndrome.

Table 1
Differential Diagnosis of Atrophy

Atrophy	LSIL	HSIL	
Cell type	Parabasal	Superficial, intertermediate	Metaplastic
Pleomorphism	+	++	+++
Nuclei	Large	Enlarged	Small
Contour	Smooth	Irregular +	Irregular ++/+++
Chromatin	Bland/smudgy	Dark+	Dark++
n:c ratio	Normal	Increased +	Increased++

+, mild; ++, moderate; +++, severe. HSIL, high-grade squamous intra-epithelial lesion; LSIL, low-grade squamous intra-epithelial lesion; n:c, nuclear-to-cytoplasmic ratio.

Table 2
Distinguishing Features of Atrophy vs Small-Cell Carcinoma

Atrophy	Small cell ca
Large sheets of cells	Fewer cells
Bland nuclei	Hyperchromatic nuclei
Regular shape of nucleus	Irregular shape
Coarse chromatin	Bland chromatin
No necrosis	Necrosis

Table 3
Diagnostic Pitfalls in Atrophy

Entities	Distinguishing features in atrophy
• Keratinizing dysplasia	Pseudokeratinization has low n:c and no Nuclear and cytoplasmic abnormalities
• HSIL	Smudgy nuclei and lack of nuclear detail
• LSIL	Uniform nuclei and lack of nuclear detail
• Invasive squamous carcinoma	Granular diathesis lacking malignant squamous cells

HSIL, high-grade squamous intra-epithelial lesion; LSIL, low-grade squamous intra-epithelial lesion; n:c, nuclear-to-cytoplasmic ratio.

- Pituitary dysfunction.
- Bilateral oophorectomy.
- Radiation or chemotherapy.

High Estrogen States
- Estrogenic phase of menstrual cycle.
- Ovarian tumors with estrogenic activity.
- Testicular feminizing syndrome.
- Congenital absence of uterus.

Table 4
Background Debris: Atrophic Vaginitis vs Squamous Carcinoma

	Atrophic vaginitis	Squamous-cell carcinoma
Background	Granular debris	Necrotic and granular debris
	Acute inflammation	Acute inflammation
		Blood
Cell type	Parabasal	All range of squamous cells
Cell shape	Polygonal	Round, spindled to bizarre
Nucleus	Uniform, smooth	Round to pleomorphic, irregular
	Mild hyperchromasia	Hyperchromasia prominent
Cytoplasm	Cyanophilic	Keratinized, dense
Mitosis	−	++

−, absent; ++, moderate.

Effects of Exogenous Hormonal Therapy

- In pregnancy, no effect.
- In postmenopausal women, parabasal cells mature to intermediate cells.

ATROPHY
Cytological Features of Atrophy

- Single and flat monolayer sheets of mature and immature parabasal and basal cells predominate.
- Enlarged pale, nuclei (three to five times the area of an intermediate cell nucleus) with smooth contours, and bland uniformly distributed chromatin.
- Slight increase in the nuclear-to-cytoplasmic (n:c) ratio.
- Focal pseudokeratinization resulting from the effect of drying and degeneration.
- "Blue blobs" (basophilic and amorphous degenerating parabasal cells).
- Granular inflammatory background debris in atrophy is similar to the necrotic diathesis seen in squamous-cell carcinoma. A diagnosis of cancer should only be made in the presence of malignant squamous cells.

Pap Smear Findings in Atrophic Vaginitis

- "Blue blobs."
- Cellularity is variable.
- Chromatin is smudgy.
- Debris.
- Polygonal-round cells with slight pleomorphism.
- Acute inflammation.
- On liquid-based preparation, clumps of granular background debris with acute inflammatory cells and apoptosis appears similar to the granular diathesis of squamous-cell carcinoma. Atrophy is distinguished from cancer by the absence of malignant squamous cells.

CHANGES SEEN ON PAP TEST IN PREGNANCY

- Navicular cells.
- Decidual cells.

- Folic acid deficiency.
- Arias–Stella reaction.
- Trophoblastic cells (Fig. 7.4).

Navicular Cells

- Glycogenated intermediate cells with a boat-like configuration also known as "navicular" cells predominate during pregnancy.

Decidual Cells (Figs. 7.5 and 7.6)

- Cervical stromal cells with decidualization may be seen during pregnancy, postpartum, and with oral contraceptive pills.
- Cells occur singly or in clusters.
- Cells are large and polygonal.
- Nuclei are large, round, degenerative, and smudged with prominent nucleoli.
- Cytoplasm is moderate in amount with lacy, pale-pink cytoplasm.
- Low n:c.
- May mimic atypical squamous cells of undetermined significance or low-grade squamous intra-epithelial lesions (Table 5).

Folic Acid Deficiency

- May occur in pregnancy or with oral contraceptive use.
- Increase in cell size, and an increase cytoplasm.
- Increase in nuclear size with occasional binucleation.
- Chromatin is delicate and uniform.
- Low n:c.
- Neutrophils show multilobation (>7 lobes).
- May mimic radiation-induced cellular changes, atypical squamous cells of undetermined significance, or low-grade squamous intra-epithelial lesions.

Arias–Stella Reaction (Figs 7.7 and 7.8)

- Proliferative changes are seen in endometrial and endocervical cells.
- Cells are large.
- Nucleus is large, hyperchromatic, and multilobated.
- Nucleoli are prominent.
- Cytoplasm is abundant and multivacuolated.
- Low n:c.
- Differential diagnosis includes endometrial and clear-cell carcinoma.
- Clinical history of pregnancy may prove helpful.

Trophoblastic Cells

- Syncytiotrophoblasts are large multinucleated cells with irregular outlines.
- Nuclei are round, regular, and hyperchromatic.
- Cytoplasm is abundant.
- Cytotrophoblasts are small and mononucleated, singly dispersed, and may mimic atypical squamous cells that cannot exclude high-grade squamous intra-epithelial lesions, or high-grade squamous intra-epithelial lesions.
- Trophoblastic cells are rarely seen in normal pregnancy.

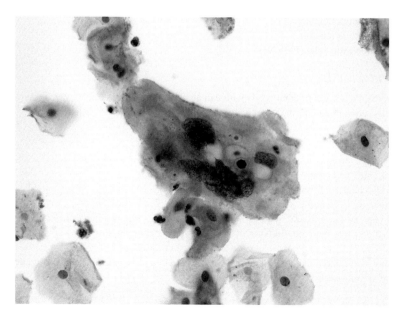

Fig. 7.4. Syncytiotrophoblast. Note giant cell (ThinPrep; Papanicolaou stain).

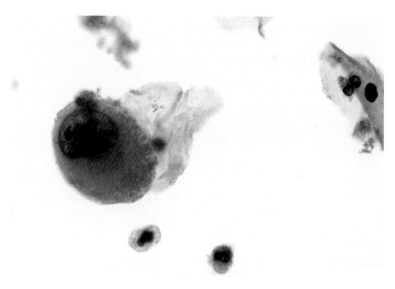

Fig. 7.5. Decidual cell (ThinPrep; Papanicolaou stain).

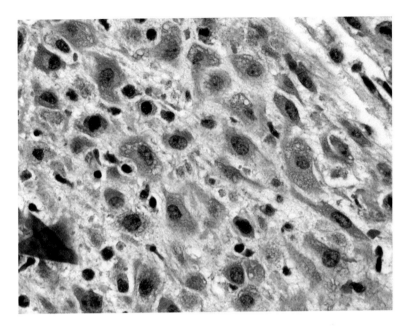

Fig. 7.6. Decidua. Same case as in Fig. 7.5 (H&E stain).

Table 5
Decidual Cells vs Low-Grade Squamous Intra-Epithelial Lesions

Features	Decidual cells	LSIL
Cytoplasm	Abundant, pale and degenerative	Mature
Koilocytosis	Absent	Present with HPV
Nuclei	Smooth contours	"Raisinoid" with HPV
Nucleolus	Prominent, basophilic	Absent
History	Helpful (pregnancy, postpartum)	May not help

Note: abundant pale cytoplasm and central round nucleus with prominent nucleoli differentiates decidual cells from LSIL.
HPV, human papillomavirus; LSIL, low-grade squamous intra-epithelial lesion.

- During the first trimester, the presence of trophoblasts may indicate an abortion.
- During the third trimester their presence may indicate placental abruption.
- During postpartum their presence may indicate retained placenta.
- Differential diagnosis of syncytiotrophoblasts include Herpes simplex virus infection and Langhans' giant cells seen in tuberculosis, low-grade squamous intra-epithelial lesion, choriocarcinoma, or another high-grade malignancy.

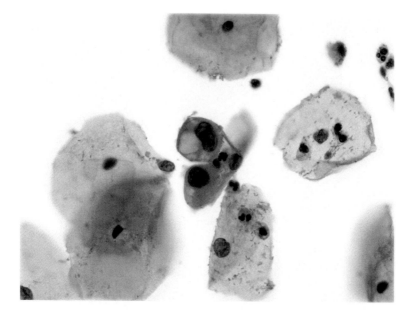

Fig. 7.7. Arias–Stella reaction (ThinPrep; Papanicolaou stain).

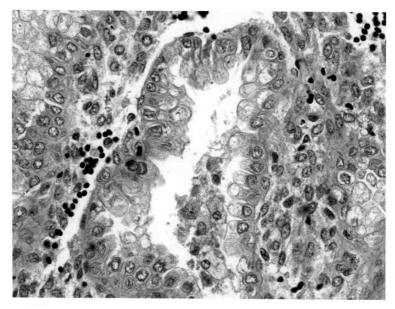

Fig. 7.8. Arias–Stella reaction. Same case as in Fig. 7.7 (H&E stain).

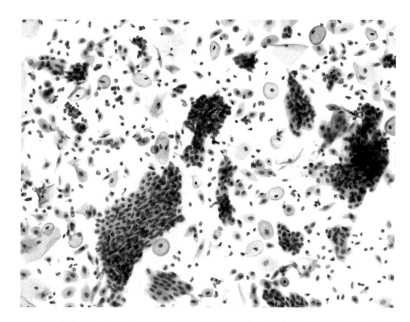

Fig. 7.9. Atrophy. Compare with Fig. 7.10 (SurePath, Papanicolaou stain).

POSTPARTUM CHANGES

- Predominantly parabasal cells resulting from the loss of the hormonal effect of pregnancy.
- Few glycogenated intermediate cells.
- Usually lasts for 6 weeks or until normal ovarian function ensues.
- Mimics atrophy (Figs. 7.9–7.18).

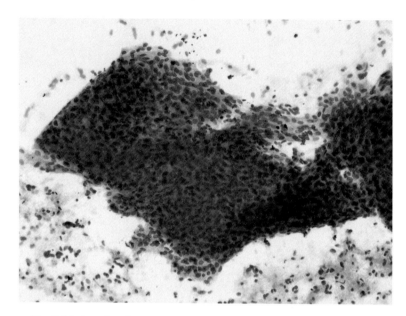

Fig. 7.10. Atrophy. Compare with Fig. 7.9 (ThinPrep, Papanicolaou stain).

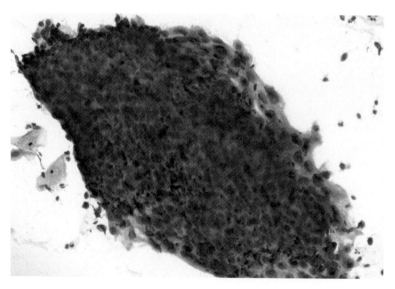

Fig. 7.11. Squamous cell carcinoma. Compare with Figs. 7.9 and 7.10 (ThinPrep, Papanicolaou stain).

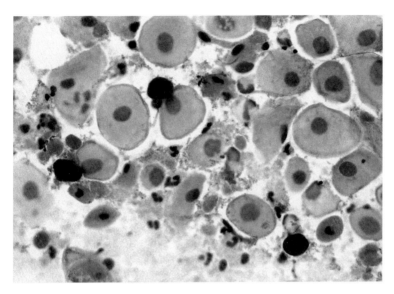

Fig. 7.12. Atrophic vaginitis, "blue-blobs," and granular background debris (conventional smear, Papanicolaou stain).

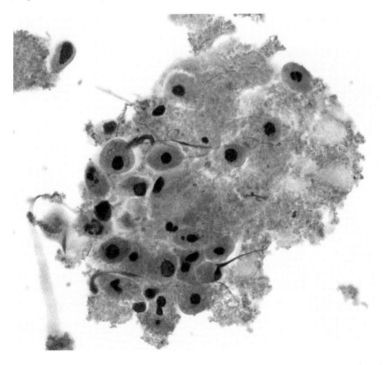

Fig. 7.13. Atrophic vaginitis. Granular background debris is similar to conventional smear in Fig. 7.12 (ThinPrep, Papanicolaou stain).

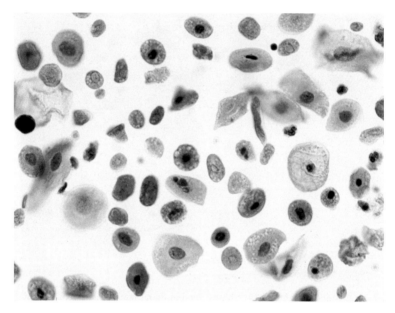

Fig. 7.14. Atrophy. Granular background debris is clumped and seen in a different plane of focus. Compare with Figs. 7.12 and 7.13 (SurePath, Papanicolaou stain).

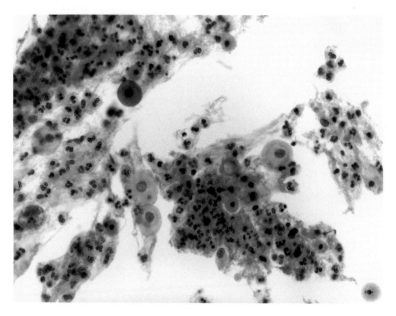

Fig. 7.15. Atrophic vaginitis, pseudokeratinized cells. Compare with Fig. 7.16 (ThinPrep, Papanicolaou stain).

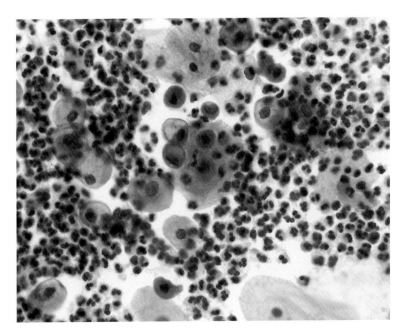

Fig. 7.16. Atrophic vaginitis, pseudokeratinized cells. Compare with Fig. 7.15 (conventional smear, Papanicolaou stain).

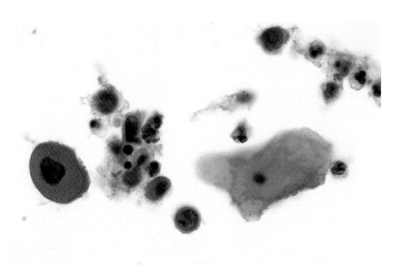

Fig. 7.17. High-grade keratinizing dysplasia. Compare with Figs. 7.15 and 7.16 (ThinPrep, Papanicolaou stain).

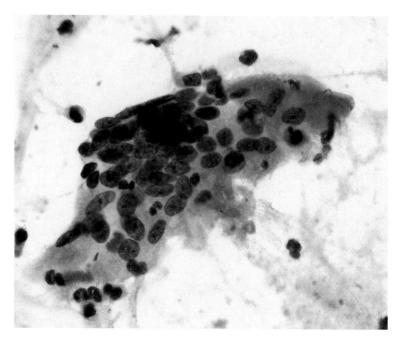

Fig. 7.18. Giant histiocytic cell in atrophy. Compare with syncytiotrophoblast in Fig. 7.4 (ThinPrep; Papanicolaou stain).

8

Reactive Changes and Organisms

INTRODUCTION

Any non-neoplastic findings and organisms in a Pap test, without cellular changes of preneoplasia or neoplasia, are mentioned under the interpretation/result category of "negative for intra-epithelial lesion or malignancy."

NONNEOPLASTIC FINDINGS

- Reactive changes associated with inflammation, repair, and intrauterine device (IUD).
- Organisms.
- Glandular cells status–post-hysterectomy.
- Atrophy.
- Other nonneoplastic findings.

Reactive Squamous Cells (Fig. 8.1)

- Nuclei enlarged (approximately two times intermediate cell nuclei), round with smooth contours, mild hyperchromasia, and eosinophilia.
- Binucleation.
- Nucleoli may be prominent.
- Cytoplasm with small perinuclear halos.
- Polychromasia.

Cytological Features of Repair and Regeneration (Fig. 8.2)

- Epithelial regeneration in response to persistent irritation.
- Two-dimensional flat cohesive sheets with no overlapping "streaming effect."
- Cells aligned in the same direction with a "school of fish appearance."
- Cells are enlarged.
- Well-defined cell borders.
- Single cells are rare.
- Low nuclear-to-cytoplasmic (n:c) ratio.
- Nuclei are enlarged and rounded with a smooth membrane, and may be multiple in number.
- Fine chromatin.
- Nucleoli are single or multiple and prominent.
- Cytoplasm is abundant, cyanophilic or polychromatic, and vacuolated.
- Mitoses present.
- Neutrophils are often present.
- May mimic neoplastic lesions.

From: *Fundamentals of Pap Test Cytology*
By: R. S. Hoda and S. A. Hoda © Humana Press Inc., Totowa, NJ

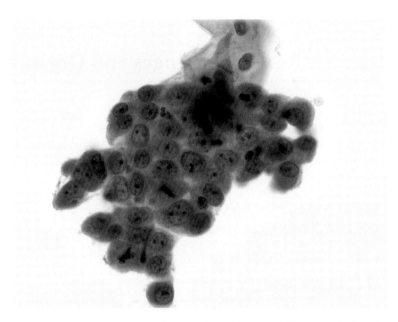

Fig. 8.1. Reactive regenerative cells. Note the uniform nuclei with nucleoli and mitoses (ThinPrep; Papanicolaou stain).

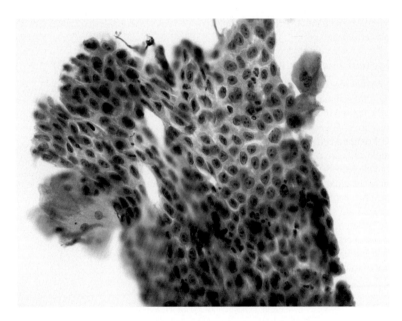

Fig. 8.2. Reactive reparative cells. Cohesive sheet of cells with "streaming" effect (SurePath; Papanicolaou stain).

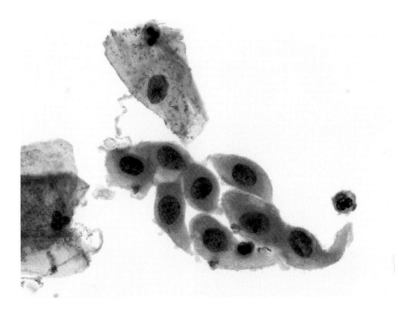

. **Fig. 8.3.** Squamous metaplastic cells. Cells show smooth nuclei and cytoplasmic extensions (ThinPrep; Papanicolaou stain).

- Liquid-based preparations (LBP) may show less "streaming" with more rounded cells.
- Polychromatic staining may be seen.

Squamous Metaplasia (Fig. 8.3)

- Reparative change is seen at the transformation zone.
- Cells are in a cobblestone arrangement.
- Nuclei are uniform and smooth with uniform fine chromatin.
- Cytoplasm is dense or vacuolated with rigid contours and elongations.

Radiation Effect (Figs. 8.4 and 8.5)

- Cells are arranged in loosely cohesive sheets.
- Cellular enlargement (macrocytosis).
- Multinucleated giant cells.
- Low n:c.
- Nuclei are markedly enlarged with smudged chromatin, and may be multiple in number.
- Nucleoli are prominent and may be multiple in number.
- Cytoplasm is abundant, vacuolated, and polychromatic.
- Background in a conventional smear is unique and shows dried mucoid and proteinaceous material in "ball-like" clumps.

Hyperkeratosis (Fig. 8.6)

- Anucleate squamous in patches.
- Site of previous nucleus is seen as a light central area.
- Caused by chronic irritation.

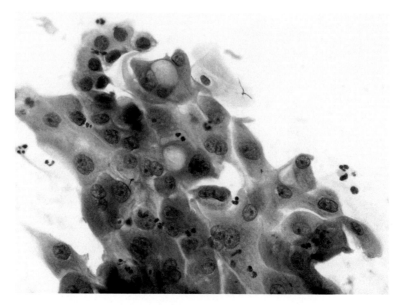

Fig. 8.4. Radiation change. Two-dimensional sheet, binucleation, cytoplasmic vacuolation, and low nuclear-to-cytoplasmic ratio (conventional smear; Papanicolaou stain).

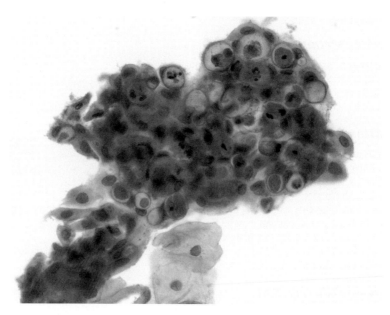

Fig. 8.5. Radiation change. Note the intracytoplasmic proteinaceous debris characteristic of therapy (ThinPrep; Papanicolaou stain).

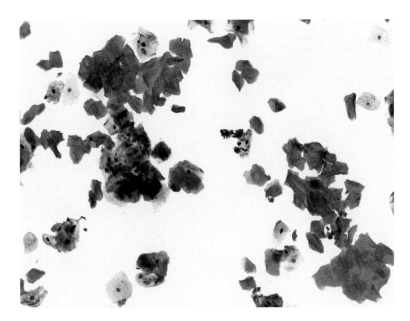

Fig. 8.6. Hyperkeratosis with plaques of anucleated squamous cells (ThinPrep; Papanicolaou stain).

- Extensive hyperkeratosis (patches of hyperkeratosis with irregular, angulated edges present in at least five ×10 fields) may indicate significant underlying pathology.

Parakeratosis (Fig. 8.7)

- Caused by chronic irritation.
- Isolated or in loose sheets.
- Miniature polygonal squamous cells.
- Nuclei are small, uniform, and pyknotic central.
- Cytoplasm is eosinophilic to orangeophilic.
- Extensive or persistent parakeratosis in a patient with a history of dysplasia may warrant close follow-up.

Reactive Endocervical Cells (Fig. 8.8)

- Cells are enlarged and distorted.
- Nuclei are enlarged, round to ovoid, and have fine chromatin.
- Nucleoli are prominent.
- Cytoplasm is vacuolated, abundant, and columnar.
- Low n:c ratio.
- Multinucleation seen in pregnancy may mimic low-grade squamous intra-epithelial lesions.
- Seen with inflammation, status–postcone biopsy, endocervical brushing.

Tubal Metaplasia (Fig. 8.9)

- May be seen in the upper third of the endocervix.
- Most common cause of atypical endocervical cells.

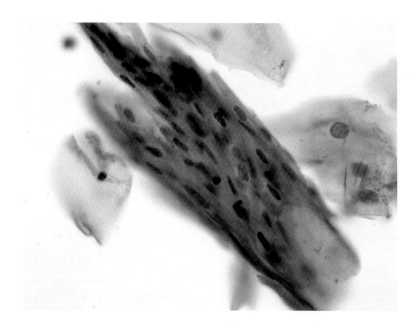

Fig. 8.7. Parakeratosis. Note uniform, small, centrally placed nuclei (ThinPrep; Papanicolaou stain).

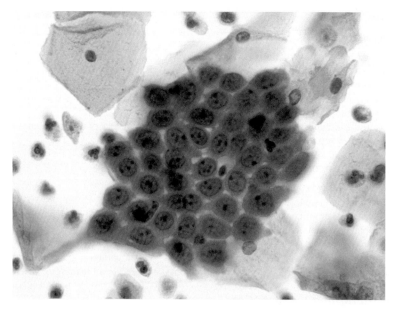

Fig. 8.8. Reactive endocervical cells in a "honeycomb" configuration (ThinPrep; Papanicolaou stain).

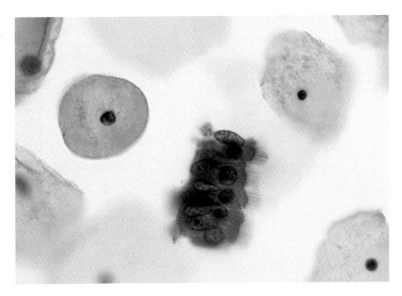

Fig. 8.9. Tubal metaplasia. Note cilia (ThinPrep; Papanicolaou stain).

- Small groups, pseudostratified strips, or crowded groups.
- Nuclei are small, round to oval, enlarged, usually centrally located, may be atypical, hyperchromatic, and nucleoli may be seen.
- Cytoplasm is columnar, may show discrete vacuoles, cilia, or terminal bar.
- Differential diagnosis includes adenocarcinoma *in situ*.
- Rare cases of ciliated endocervical adenocarcinoma have been reported.

Microglandular Hyperplasia (Fig. 8.10)

- Benign endocervical proliferation.
- Associated with oral contraceptive use.
- Morphologically, microglandular hyperplasia has a glandular or metaplastic pattern.
- Glandular pattern shows three-dimensional clusters of cells with microlumina and fenestrations, nuclei are enlarged and may be atypical, nuclear grooves and nucleoli are present, cytoplasm shows prominent vacuoles, cilia and "feathering" is not seen, cytological features may overlap those of atypical glandular cells or adenocarcinoma.
- Metaplastic pattern has groups of cells with hyperchromatic and smudgy nuclei with grooves; cytological features may overlap those of atypical squamous cells that cannot exclude atypical squamous cells of undetermined significance and high-grade squamous intra-epithelial lesion (HSIL).
- Negative immunostaining with carcinoembryonic antigen is confirmatory of the benign nature of the lesion.

IUD-Related Changes (Fig. 8.11)

- Changes are seen in endometrial or endocervical cells.
- Endometrial cells may be shed at midcycle.

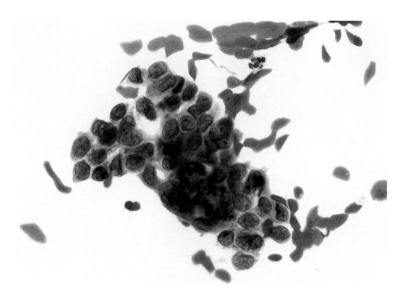

Fig. 8.10. Microglandular hyperplasia, metaplastic type (ThinPrep; Papanicolaou stain).

- Cells are single or in small clusters.
- High n:c.
- Nuclei are uniform with slight hyperchromasia and prominent nucleoli.
- Cytoplasm is abundant with large secretory vacuoles.
- May mimic an endometrial adenocarcinoma. Clinical history of IUD use may be helpful.
- Single IUD cells may mimic HSIL. The presence of rare, atypical cells and lack of nuclear membrane irregularity and chromatin changes help distinguish these cells from HSIL.
- *Actinomyces* is associated with IUD use in 25% of cases.
- Calcified debris seen with IUD may mimic psammoma bodies.

Follicular Cervicitis (Fig. 8.12)

- Aggregates of benign polymorphous lymphocytes with actual germinal center formation.
- Tingible body macrophages.
- Inflammatory cells.
- Dirty background.
- Capillaries traversing lymphoid aggregates.
- Approximately 50% of patients have chlamydial infection.
- May be mistaken for malignant lymphoma.
- On LBP, the lymphoid cells may appear in clusters and may be mistaken for endometrial-type cells.

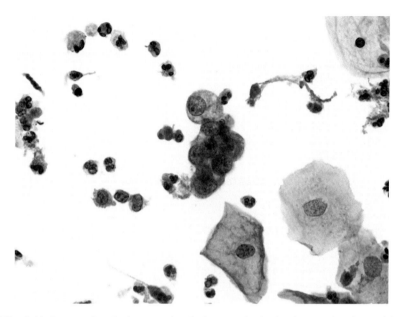

Fig. 8.11. Intrauterine device-associated changes. A single cluster of endometrial cells with vacuolated cytoplasm (ThinPrep; Papanicolaou stain).

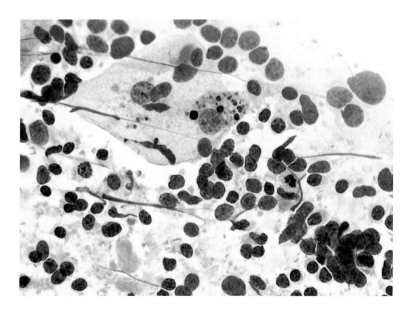

Fig. 8.12. Follicular cervicitis shows lymphoid cells and a tingible-body macrophage (conventional smear; Papanicolaou stain).

Transitional Cell Metaplasia

- Cohesive fragments with multilayering and streaming.
- Nuclei are oval to elongated with longitudinal grooves, wrinkled contour, fine chromatin, and small or inconspicuous nucleoli.
- May mimic HSIL.

Pseudoparakeratosis

- May be related to oral contraceptive use.
- Eosinophilic or orangeophilic staining of glandular cell cytoplasm.
- May mimic HSIL.

Cytomorphology of Histiocytes in Pap Smears

- Single cells of variable size.
- Oval shape.
- Bean-shaped nucleus that may be multinucleated.
- Large nucleolus.
- Well-defined cytoplasm with phagocytized material.
- Cytoplasmic vacuoles and granular cytoplasm.
- May mimic HSIL or endometrial epithelial cells.

Benign Glandular Cells Status Post-Total Hysterectomy

- Cells may be glandular-, metaplastic-, or parabasal-type cells.
- Seen in approx 2% of vaginal Pap tests, mostly from women with a history of prior radiation therapy for malignancy.
- May represent a metaplastic change in vaginal mucosa or cells from a vaginal inclusion cyst resulting from trauma or Gartner's duct cyst, or vaginal adenosis not associated with diethylstilbestrol.
- Frequently occur in groups.
- Intracytoplasmic mucin may be seen either diffusely or with cytoplasmic vacuoles.
- If the cells look perfectly benign, they can be categorized either as benign glandular cells or as reactive cellular changes to avoid aggressive follow-up.

ORGANISMS SEEN IN PAP TEST INCLUDE (TABLE 1)

- Bacterial: *Gardnerella vaginalis*, *Actinomyces*, *Neisseria gonorrhea*, *Chlamydia trachomatis*.
- Viral: Human papillomavirus, herpes simplex virus (HSV), cytomegalovirus (CMV), *Molluscum contagiosum*.
- Fungal: *Candida* spp.
- Parasites: *Trichomonas vaginalis*, *Entamoeba histolytica*.

Diagnostic Terms Used for Organisms in the Bethesda System

- *T. vaginalis*.
- Fungal organisms morphologically consistent with *Candida* spp.
- Shift in vaginal flora suggestive of bacterial vaginosis.
- Cellular changes consistent with herpes.
- Microorganisms morphologically consistent with *Actinomyces* spp.

Note: Bacterial vaginosis, *Actinomyces*, and definitive characterization of *Candida* spp. may require microbiological culture or immunological assay.

Table 1
Features of Various Infections Observed on the Pap Test

Actinomyces	Long, branching filamentous bacteria—often in tangled clumps "Gupta bodies."
Candida	Yeasts and pseudohyphae
CMV	Characteristic nuclear and cytoplasmic inclusions surrounded by a pale halo.
Bacterial	Seen as "clue" cells, squamous cells covered by small vaginosis coccobacillary forms.
Herpes	Large, multinucleated, ground-glass nuclei with molding.
Leptothrix	Long, filamentous bacterium; thread-like.
Normal flora	*Lactobacilli*, rod-shaped, Gram-positive, blue on Pap stain.
Trichomonas	Pear-shaped, red, cytoplasmic granules with a narrow nucleus.

Trichomonas (Figs. 8.13 and 8.14)

- Most common parasitic infection of the female genital tract.
- 15–30 μm.
- Small, round-to-oval "pear-shaped" organisms with an indistinct eccentric nucleus and red cytoplasmic granules.
- Stains gray-blue.
- Dirty, fuzzy background with round aggregates of neutrophils ("cannonballs" or "pus ball").
- Reactive nuclear changes, perinuclear halos, and pseudoeosinophilia of the cytoplasm and the nucleus.
- Leptothrix is associated with *T. vaginalis* in approx 80% of cases.
- Cytoplasmic fragments from degenerating squamous or glandular cells may mimic trichomonads.
- On LBP eosinophilic granules better visualized and flagella are preserved.

Leptothrix (Fig. 8.14)

- Form of *lactobacillus*.
- Appear as diffusely scattered long, filamentous "hair-like" rods.
- Commonly associated with *Trichomonas*.

Candida *spp. (Fig. 8.15)*

- Most common species are *Candida albicans* and *Candida glabrata*.
- *C. albicans* shows nonseptated pseudohyphae and budding yeast forms.
- *C. glabrata* consists of small, uniform, round, budding yeast forms surrounded by clear halos. No pseudohyphal forms are seen in vivo or in culture.
- Reactive changes in squamous cells comprise of slight nuclear enlargement, small perinuclear halos, and nucleoli.
- Pseudokeratinization or eosinophilia of squamous cells.
- Heavy accompanying inflammation.
- *Candida* hyphae should be distinguished from *Trichophyton*, which may present as a contaminant in the Pap test. *Trichophyton* are septate with branching.
- On LBP, *Candida* also shows a "shish-kebab" appearance with squamous cells "skewered" through fungal pseudohyphae.

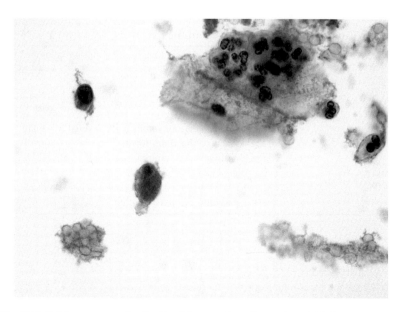

Fig. 8.13. *Trichomonas vaginalis.* Grayish, pear-shaped organism (ThinPrep; Papanicolaou stain).

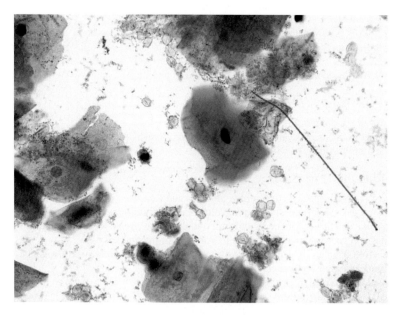

Fig. 8.14. Leptothrix and *Trichmonas vaginalis* occasionally coexist (ThinPrep; Papanicolaou stain).

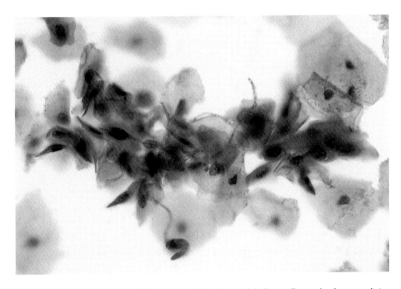

Fig. 8.15. *Candida* spp. with "shish-kebab" effect (ThinPrep; Papanicolaou stain).

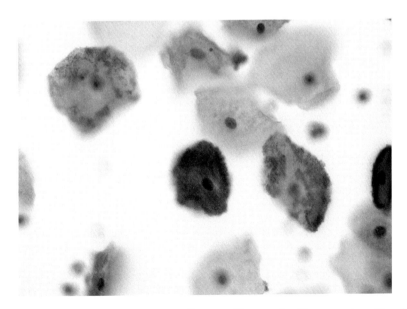

Fig. 8.16. "Clue cells" are squamous cells covered by coccobacillary organisms (SurePath; Papanicolaou stain).

Bacterial Vaginosis (Fig. 8.16)

- Complex vaginal infection that results from loss of normal vaginal bacterial flora (*lactobacilli*).
- Fairly common and affects millions of women annually.
- Previously attributed solely to *G. vaginalis*; however, recent studies implicate other bacteria, as well as many newly recognized species including three bacteria in the *Clostridiales* order.
- Many women with bacterial vaginosis are asymptomatic, and many others only have a malodorous vaginal discharge.
- May be associated with several adverse health affects including preterm labor, pelvic inflammatory disease, and low birth weight.
- Clinical diagnosis is based on four features including:
  - Thin, milky vaginal discharge.
  - pH greater than 4.5.
  - Positive "whiff test" (production of a fishy odor when 10% potassium hydroxide is added to a slide with vaginal fluid from the patient).
  - "Clue cells" on wet prep.

Diagnosis is confirmed when at least three of these criteria are present.

- "Clue cells" are characteristic of bacterial vaginosis and represent squamous cells covered with numerous *coccobacilli*.
- Cytological criteria include, "clue cells," absence of *lactobacilli*, scanty neutrophils, and profuse-free *coccibacilli* scattered among cornified-type epithelial cells.
- Responds to empirical antibiotic therapy.

Herpes Simplex Virus (Fig. 8.17)

- Causes herpetic keratitis, encephalitis, and vaginitis.
- Multinucleation, ground-glass nuclei with molding, thick nuclear membranes because of margination of chromatin, and eosinophilic intranuclear inclusions.
- Should be distinguished from multinucleated endocervical cells.
- Although easily detected on cytology, immunochemistry may be used in equivocal cases.
- Recently, *in situ* hybridization and polymerase chain reaction amplification (on destained Pap smears) have increasingly been used for the detection of HSV because of an increase in specificity and sensitivity, and in cases with poorly preserved or few HSV cells.
- The specificity and sensitivity of *in situ* hybridization compared with immunochemistry is 100 vs 85% and 94 vs 74%, respectively.

Actinomyces (Figs. 8.18 and 8.19)

- Infection may be asymptomatic or consist of a foul-smelling vaginal discharge containing sulfur granules.
- Associated with IUD usage.
- Gram-positive bacteria.
- Tangled clusters of grayish-blue filamentous bacterial colonies with acute angle branching (Gupta bodies) and dense center. This pattern is seen on both conventional smears and LBP.
- On LBP, in addition to this morphology, the filamentous nature is more clearly visualized. The organisms may also be arranged as horizontal array of filamentous structures along a central core, probably representing part of the IUD strings. They appear dense toward the inner portion of the array.
- Infection is accompanied by marked inflammatory infiltrate of polymorphonuclear neutrophils, macrophages, and rare multinucleated giant cells.

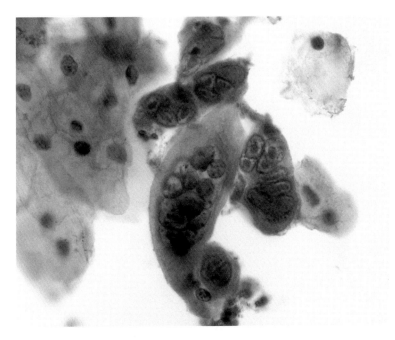

Fig. 8.17. Herpesvirus. Multinucleated cells with nuclear molding and eosinophilic nuclear inclusions (ThinPrep; Papanicolaou stain).

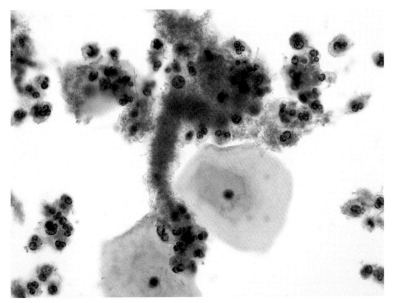

Fig. 8.18. *Actinomyces* organisms on liquid-based cytology appear fine and filamentous, sometimes arranged in a transverse array along a central core probably representing part of the intrauterine device strings (ThinPrep; Papanicolaou stain).

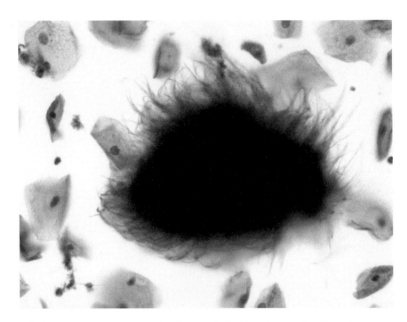

Fig. 8.19. *Actinomyces* seen as the characteristic "dust bunnies" with a dense center surrounded by delicate filaments radiating from the central condensation ("Gupta bodies.") This appearance is also seen on conventional smears (SurePath; Papanicolaou stain).

Table 2
Reactive Inflammatory Atypia vs Dysplasia

	Atypia from inflammation	Dysplasia
Cells	Single/loose clusters	Same
Nuclear size	2 × Normal intermediate. Nucleus	<3 × Normal interm. nucleus
Nucleus	Regular contour	Irregular contour
	Chromatin dark, even	Chromatin dark, irregular
Nucleoli	+	–
Cytoplasm	May have vacuoles	May be denser
	Cell membrane indistinct	Cell membrane distinct
	Altered staining	–
	Perinuclear halos +	–
N:c ratio	Normal	Increase +/++
Background	Generally exudative	Generally nonexudative

Cytomegalovirus

- DNA virus of the Herpes family.
- Can be seen in immunocompetent and immunocompromised patients.
- May cause endocervicitis and is rarely seen on a Pap smear.
- Cytomegaly and karyomegaly.
- Prominent, cherry-red intranuclear inclusions surrounded by a halo.

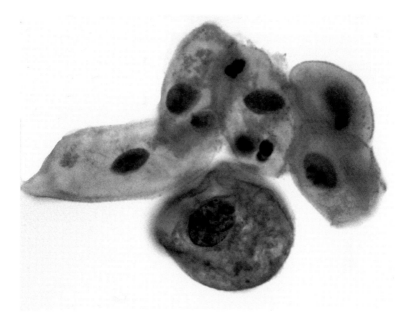

Fig. 8.20. Reactive nonspecific inflammatory changes which may mimic atypical squamous cells of undetermined significance (ThinPrep; Papanicolaou stain).

Table 3
Reactive Inflammatory Atypia vs Glandular Atypia

	Inflammatory atypia	Glandular atypia
Cells	Single/sheets	Single/aggregates
Shape of cells	Variable	Columnar
Nucleus	Normochromic	Hyperchromatic
Nucleoli	Macronucleoli	Less prominent
Cytoplasm	Granular, goblet cells	Less granular
Background	Generally exudative	Generally nonexudative
Mitoses	+	+
Apoptosis	−	+
Diathesis	Nontumoral	Tumoral

- Basopholic cytoplasmic inclusions.
- Immunocytochemical positivity of the nuclei and perinuclear cytoplasmic inclusions is confirmatory.

Inflammatory Changes That Mimic Atypical Cells (Tables 2 and 3; Fig. 8.20)

- Nuclear enlargement.
- Perinuclear halo may appear bigger and vaguely resemble a koilocyte.

Characteristic Infectious Inclusions Seen in Pap Smears

- Human papillomavirus: perinuclear cytoplasmic clearing (koilocytes).
- Herpesvirus: intranuclear, ground-glass inclusions.
- CMV: intranuclear: single, large, round.
  intracytoplasmic: multiple, small.

9

Human Papillomavirus in Cervical Carcinogenesis

- Cervical carcinoma is the second most common cancer in women worldwide, affecting more than 400,000 women annually, breast carcinoma being the first.
- In the United States in 2005 there were approx 10,500 new cases of cervical cancer, and approx 3900 women died of the disease.
- The majority of squamous cancers are preceded by premalignant lesions, which may persist for decades. The premalignant lesion sheds cells that can be detected in the Pap test. This test has led to a 70% decline in the incidence of cervical carcinoma over the last 60 years.
- Epidemiological and molecular studies have shown that high-risk human papillomavirus (HPV) is the main causative agent of invasive squamous-cell carcinoma.
- Cervical HPV is detected in 5–40% of asymptomatic women of reproductive age, 50–75% of which are high-risk type. The majority of these infections are transient and only show minor cytological abnormalities consisting of koilocytes or low-grade squamous intra-epithelial lesion (LSIL). However, some infections caused by certain high-risk HPV types may persist and ultimately progress to cervical intra-epithelial neoplasia 3/carcinoma *in situ* (CIN 3/CIS, high-grade squamous intra-epithelial lesion 3 [HSIL3]). Less than half of HPV infections persist for 2 years or more. Persistent infections are defined as amounts of HPV DNA sufficient enough to be detected using standard molecular techniques.
- Overall, approx 20 million Americans (15% of the population) are infected with HPV.
- Approximately 6.2 million Americans acquire a new genital infection every year.
- Resulting from a greater understanding of the biological nature and oncogenic potential of various high-risk HPV types, the HPV test is currently being used with cytology screening to improve disease detection.

TYPES OF HPV

- More than 100 different types of HPV have been identified and each is known by a number.
- About 30 types of HPV infect the genital tract and one-third of these have a potential to lead to invasive squamous cancer (Table 1).
- Genital HPV is subdivided into low-risk (6, 11, 42–44, 54, 61, 70, 72, and 81) and high-risk types (16, 18, 31, 33, 35, 39, 45, 51, 52, 56, 58, 59, 61, 66, 68, 73, and 82).
- Low-risk HPV usually causes benign proliferative lesions, such as condyloma acuminata, the most common type of sexually transmitted disease. HPV 6 and 11 are the ones most frequently associated with genital warts. Rarely, low-risk HPV have been associated with invasive squamous cancer.
- High-risk types are associated with lesions that are at a high risk for malignant progression, particularly in the anogenital tract.

From: *Fundamentals of Pap Test Cytology*
By: R. S. Hoda and S. A. Hoda © Humana Press Inc., Totowa, NJ

Table 1
HPV: Types, Oncogenic Potential, and Lesions Caused

Risk	HPV types	Lesions
Low	6, 11, 40, 42–44, 53, 54, 61, 72, 73, and 81	Condyloma, LSIL
High[a]	16, 18, 31, 33, 35, 39, 45, 51, 52, 56, 58, 59, 68, and 82	LSIL, HSIL, carcinoma

[a]High-risk types 16, 18, 31, and 45 cause the majority (80%) of cervical cancers.
HSIL, high-grade squamous intra-epithelial lesion; LSIL, low-grade squamous intra-epithelial lesion.

- Certain viral subtypes of high-risk HPV are much more commonly associated with cancer than other subtypes, including HPV 16 and 18, which are found in more than 70% of cervical cancers.

NATURE AND MOLECULAR STRUCTURE OF HPV

- Analysis of HPV is performed by molecular hybridization techniques on DNA extracted from tissues and cells.
- HPV is a member of the Papillomaviridae family of DNA viruses.
- It is epitheliotropic and mucosotropic.
- HPV is a double-stranded DNA virus, measures 55 nm in diameter, and consists of a protein capsid that is icoshedral and encloses a circular genome.
- The circular genome consists of 7900 base pairs, encodes eight viral proteins, and is divisible into three regions: an early (E) region, a late (L) region, and a noncoding region. The E region codes for nonstructural proteins (*E1*, *E2*, *E6*, and *E7*) and are exressed early. *E1* is the viral replication protein. *E2* is the major viral regulator of transcription and replication. It interacts with *E1* in initiating replication and controls transcription by binding to specific sites in the viral regulatory region. The L region codes for viral capsid proteins (*L1* and *L2*) and are expressed late in viral life. The noncoding region (also known as the upstream regulatory region) contains the viral promoter, the origin of HPV replication, amongst others.
- *E2* controls the viral oncogenes, *E6* and *E7*, which play the most significant role in oncogenesis. *E6* and *E7* encode proteins capable of inducing cellular proliferation.
- Molecular analyses of condylomas and HPV-associated carcinomas have shown differences that may pertain to the differing transforming activity of these viruses.
- HPV infection may follow one of the three courses:
  - The viral DNA may stabilize in an inactive, episomal form and remain clinically latent.
  - The virus may persist in an episomal form within the host cell nucleus, replicate, and produce new viral particles. This is clinically evident as a condyloma, and cytologically as an optically clear cytoplasmic cavity (koilocytes) in the infected cells.
  - In early stages of cancer, viral DNA is integrated into the human genome with disruption of the circular genomic structure and E2 regulatory region. Loss of *E2* function allows overexpression of viral oncoproteins *E6* and *E7*. *E6* and *E7* disrupt the cell cycle by promoting the degradation of two key cell cycle regulatory proteins, the tumor suppressor genes *p53* and retinoblastoma gene (*pRb*). *E6* binds *p53* and *E7* to the *pRb*, directly stimulating and maintaining cell division and thus causing genomic instability that may lead to HSIL and cancer.
    - *E6/E7* from low-risk HPV shows a much weaker association with *pRb* and *p53*.

TROPISM OF HPV INFECTION

- HPV types that involve the anogenital tract target the keratinized squamous epithelial cells of skin and mucous membranes of the cervix, vagina, and rectum.

MODE OF HPV TRANSMISSION

- Cumulative evidence suggests mode of transmission is sexual.

RISK FACTORS ASSOCIATED WITH HPV

- Early onset of sexual activity.
- Multiple partners.
- Young age.
- Race: rates are higher in African Americans and Hispanics.
- Cigarette smoking.
- Coexisting microbial infections such as herpes simplex virus.
- Altered immune status.
- Dietary deficiencies.
- Oral contraceptives.

NATURAL HISTORY OF HPV

- In women under age 30, HPV infections are usually transient and spontaneously regress within 2–3 years.
- Multiple HPV types are detected in 20–30% of those infected.
- Prevalence of HPV peaks at 18–25 years of age, and then declines.
- 15% of HSIL may progress to invasive cancer. Although the process may take decades, HSIL should be treated.
- Persistence of HPV infection or progression to cancer depends on the severity of infection.

MOLECULAR TECHNIQUES FOR HPV DNA TESTING

High-risk HPV is now recognized as the primary causal factor in the development of cervical cancer; studies show that high-risk HPV types were found in greater than 99.7% of cervical cancer cases. However, of the approx 50 million Pap tests performed in this country, only about 3.5 million are abnormal. Only few of these are caused by high-risk viruses that have the potential of persisting and progressing to squamous-cell carcinoma. Finding these few abnormal cases is like "looking for a needle in a haystack." HPV cannot be reliably cultured in a laboratory because its replication is tightly linked to squamous cells differentiation with capsids being produced only in terminally differentiated squamous cells; thus, HPV testing relies on molecular techniques to detect high-risk HPV types to identify patients at risk for malignant progression.

Molecular techniques currently used for HPV DNA detection are:

- Amplified methods
  - Signal amplification.
    - The Hybrid Capture® 2 (hc2) HPV DNA Assay (Digene Corp., Gaithersburg, MD).
  - Target amplification.
    - Polymerase chain reaction (PCR).

- Nonamplified methods
  - The Southern blot hybridization

In situ hybridization (ISH; Ventana Medical System offers InForm HPV).

Hybrid Capture 2 (hc2) HPV DNA Assay

- The Digene hc2 HPV DNA test is the only FDA-approved HPV DNA test commercially available for clinical use.
- The hc2 HPV test uses signal amplification to detect HPV DNA.
- The hc2 is standardized and highly reproducible with a sensitivity equivalent to that of PCR technique (please *see* PCR) for accurate assessment of patient risk for CIN and carcinoma.
- Hc2 is approved for use in:
  - Primary adjunctive screening of women 30 years of age and older in conjunction with a Pap for detection of high-risk HPV to guide patient management.
  - Reflex HPV test for triage of women, of any age, with a Pap reported as atypical squamous cells of undetermined significance (ASC-US).
- The assay uses two different highly specific RNA probe cocktails to test for, either or both, low-risk and high-risk HPV types. The high-risk probe cocktail identifies HPV types 16, 18, 31, 33, 35, 39, 45, 51, 52, 56, 58, 59, and 68, and the low-risk probe mixture identifies HPV types 6, 11, 42, 43, and 44.
- Samples that can be tested include specimens collected with Hybrid Capture Cervical Sampler (hc2 DNA collection device), biopsies collected in Digene's specimen transport medium, and ThinPrep® (Cytyc Corp., Marlborough, MA) cervical cytology specimens collected in PreservCyt, including the residual sample after a ThinPrep Pap test slide has been prepared. SurePath (TriPath Inc., Burlington, NC) is not FDA approved for use in the hc2 test. However, some laboratories use it for a HPV DNA test (off-label) after independent validation.

Steps of the hc2 HPV DNA Test

The test is a five-part process, taking 6–7 hours with 2.5 hours of full technician's attention. Ninety samples can be processed together on one microtiter plate. No special specimen preparation is necessary and the assay is not subject to contamination.

- ***Denature the DNA:*** The patient sample is combined with an extraction buffer to release and denature the target DNA.
- ***Probe mixing and hybridization:*** The released target DNA is then hybridized with a specific RNA probe mixture creating RNA:DNA hybrids.
- ***Hybrid capture:*** The resultant RNA:DNA hybrids are then captured onto the surface of a microplate coated with anti-RNA:DNA antibodies.
- ***Detection for labeling:*** The bound hybrids are then reacted with a hybrid antibody linked to alkaline phosphatase, and is detected with a chemiluminiscent substrate.
- ***Detection and reporting:*** As the chemiluminiscent substrate is cleaved by the bound alkaline phosphatase, light is emitted that is measured on a luminometer in relative light units. Positive controls are used. The amount of chemiluminiscence is proportional to the amount of target DNA present in the specimen.
- Results of hc2 test are reported as positive or negative.
- The FDA-approved cutoff for a positive test result is 1.0 pg HPV DNA/mL, which corresponds to approx 5000 copies of HPV DNA.

- ◦ *Note*: The cutoff of 1 pg HPV DNA/mL is highly sensitive for identifying women at risk for HSIL (CIN 2, 3) and cancer.
- Retesting by using the retesting algorithm is recommended for test results close to the cutoff level.

SPECIMEN TYPES FOR THE hc2 TEST

- Specimens collected with a hc2 DNA collection device, biopsies collected in Digene's specimen transport medium, and ThinPrep specimens collected in PreservCyt, including the residual sample after a ThinPrep Pap test slide has been prepared.

ADVANTAGES OF THE hc2 TEST

- The sensitivity of hc2 is similar to that of PCR-based assays. It has the sensitivity to detect 1 pg HPV (about 5000 copies) per mL sample.
- No special specimen preparation is necessary.
- Assay is not subject to contamination.

DISADVANTAGE OF THE hc2 TEST

- Although the assay allows one to differentiate between high- and low-risk types of HPV, individual HPV types cannot be identified without the purchase of additional special reagents.

Polymerase Chain Reaction

PCR is a technique that is used to amplify a specific region of DNA to produce an adequate amount that can be tested for HPV using hybridization techniques. PCR is the most common target-amplified technique to identify HPV DNA. It is ideal for use on specimens with low DNA content, as it has the capacity to produces highly concentrated samples of a specific DNA genetic sequence even from little viral DNA (10–100 ng). The amplification of DNA is produced by multiple, automated thermal cycles of in vitro DNA synthesis using type-specific DNA primer sets. The primers are of two types—type-specific primers that target E6/E7 region and consensus primers that amplify a conserved region in L1. Strict laboratory procedures are required to prevent contamination.

Steps in PCR

- In order to use PCR, the exact sequence of nucleotides that flank both ends of the region of DNA to be amplified must be known. This is determined by using gel electrophoresis. The primers used must be duplicates of these nucleotide sequences.
- The target DNA is heated, which denatures the DNA resulting in two single strands.
- This is followed by hybridization of the target DNA with HPV-specific primers.
- Most PCR methods utilize "consensus" primers, and the two most common primer sets are MY09/MY11 and GP5+GP6. The primers bind to their complimentary bases on the now single-stranded DNA.
- The amplification of DNA is then produced by multiple, automated thermal cycles of in vitro DNA synthesis that uses a thermostable DNA polymerase.
- Each cycle consists of primer extension, denaturation, and reannealing.
- The cycle can be repeated 20–30 times. Twenty cycles will theoretically produce approx 1 million copies of the original sequence.

- The amplified DNA can then be further analyzed to determine specific HPV types. This can be achieved either by direct visualization on gels (Southern blot) or detected by specific probes using traditional hybridization methods.

SPECIMEN TYPE FOR PCR

- Liquid-based cytology, conventional smears, fresh, and fixed tissue.

ADVANTAGES OF PCR

- Extremely sensitive and specific.
- The PCR method using primer sets, MY09/MY11 and GP5+GP6, can identify HPV DNA in more than 90% of pathologically confirmed squamous intra-epithelial lesions and cancer.
- Can be performed on very small amounts of DNA (10–100 ng), and is ideal for use on specimens with low DNA content.
- Ability to determine the specific type of HPV present in a sample.

DISADVANTAGES OF PCR

- Requires considerable skills and equipment.
- Costly and thus not applicable in large cervical cancer screening programs in low-resource settings.
- Contamination of the sample: sample may be contaminated with extraneous genetic material that could generate numerous copies of irrelevant DNA leading to erroneous conclusions.

Southern Blot Hybridization

Southern blot is an important research tool and is generally used for newly identified HPV types.

Steps of Southern Blot

- The HPV genome is extracted from a specimen and is cleaved into fragments using restriction enzymes recognizing specific DNA sequences.
- The resultant fragments of double-stranded DNA are electrophoresed to separate the fragments based on their size.
- The DNA fragments are transferred to a nitrocellulose filter.
- The filter is incubated with radiolabeled type-specific HPV DNA or RNA probes that document the presence of viral DNA in a given sample.

Specimen Types of Southern Blot

- Fresh tissue.

ADVANTAGES OF SOUTHERN BLOT

- Reliably identifies specific HPV types with its combination of hybridization and restriction fragment analysis, i.e., whether HPVs are independent (episomal) or integrated into the cellular genome.

DISADVANTAGES OF SOUTHERN BLOT

- Requires large amounts of DNA.
- Labor intensive, time consuming, and requires technical expertise.
- Not reproducible.
- Relies on multiple type-specific, radioisotope-labeled probes.
- Issues concerning storing and handling of radioactive probes.

- No commercial kit available.
- Process in entirely lab based.

In Situ *Hybridization*

ISH is not FDA approved for detection of HPV DNA in cervical samples.

It allows the detection and localization of specific nucleic acid sequences directly within a cell or tissue. ISH is the only method that permits direct visualization of the virus in a morphological context.

Steps for ISH

- The procedure requires DNA or RNA probes of known types of viruses.
- The probes can be radioactive (labeled with tritium or sulfur 35) or nonradioactive (biotinylated or flouresceinated).
- The labeled HPV DNA or RNA probes are hybridized with the tissue or cytological samples.
- If target DNA is present, the labeled probes hybridize to the tissue. The hybridization process is visualized using a variety of methods, such as antibodies directed against small molecules that are attached to the DNA or RNA probes.

SPECIMEN TYPES FOR ISH

- Cytological specimens or tissue preparations.

ADVANTAGES OF ISH

- ISH maintains the morphology of the tissue being tested.
- Permits the localization of HPV DNA within cells, and allows the comparison of the morphological effects of various types of HPV.
- It is useful in differentiating cervical lesions that contain HPV 6/11 from those that contain HPV 16 or other types with oncogenic potential.
- Commercial kits are available.

DISADVANTAGE OF ISH

- Only moderate sensitivity for HPV.

CLINICAL APPLICATIONS OF HPV TESTS

Primary Adjunctive Screening: DNAwithPap™ Test

- Clinicians can request a Pap test and a high-risk HPV test at the same time to assess the risk for cervical cancer in a woman 30 years of age or older. The test is FDA-approved and called The Digene DNAwithPap test.
- The American College of Obstetricians and Gynecologists has recommended the use of this.
- The American College of Obstetricians and Gynecologists has two recommendations for screening women 30 years or older:
  ○ Testing with cervical cytology alone in those women who have had three consecutive negative Pap results on annual cervical cytology tests. They may be rescreened with cervical cytology alone every 2–3 years.

The combined use of a cervical cytology test and Digene DNAwithPap test for high-risk types of HPV. If a woman tests negative for both tests she should be rescreened with the combined tests no more frequently than every 3 years. If only one of the tests is negative, however, more frequent screening will be necessary.

- Annual gynecological examinations, including pelvic exams, are still recommended regardless of the cervical cancer screening intervals.
- More frequent cervical screening may be required for higher risk women who are immuno-compromised, including those that are HIV positive, posttransplantation, exposed to diethylstilbestrol *in utero*, or those with a previous diagnosis of cervical cancer.
- When used together, the sensitivity for HSIL and cancer can reach as high as 100%. Thus, women with negative concurrent test results can be reassured that their risk of unidentified HSIL (CIN 2, 3) or cervical cancer is approx 1 in 1000.
- The negative predictive value of these two tests for HSIL (CIN 2, 3) is 99 to 100%.

The Digene HPV Test has a **sensitivity** of more than 96% for the detection of HSIL and cancer when performed with cytology, vs 84.4% for liquid cytology alone, and 57.7% for the conventional Pap alone. This high sensitivity, combined with a very high negative predictive value, means that with negative test results the confidence that CIN 2, 3 and cancer are not present, and that the patient is not at risk for developing cervical cancer within the next several years is high.

DNAwithPap test is not intended to substitute for regular Pap screening, it is not intended to screen women younger than 30 who have normal Pap tests, it does not distinguish between HPV types or infection with more than one type or persistence of any one type, and its use has not been evaluated in women with prior abnormal Pap history or those with other risk factors, such as HIV.

Reflex HPV Test

- The reflex HPV test is performed on Pap tests reported as ASC-US.
- Equivocal-category ASC-US is the most frequently reported Pap abnormality.
- The indeterminate reporting of ASC-US on Pap is much more common than HSIL (2.5 million vs 300,000).
- Current management guidelines for ASC-US include:
  ○ Repeat Pap test with Paps at 6- and 12-month intervals and immediate colposcopy with biopsy if an abnormality is seen.
  ○ Reflex HPV testing for high-risk HPV types.
- The consensus guidelines for Reflex HPV test were published in 2002 after the ASCUS/LSIL Triage Study showed that the test is a viable option for ASC-US Paps.
- Reflex HPV test is gaining acceptance among clinicians as the most cost-effective follow-up of ASC-US Paps.

Reflex HPV Test Algorithm

- If high-risk HPV test is negative, repeat Pap in 6 months; if repeat Pap is normal, return to routine screening.
- If positive for high-risk HPV perform colposcopy.

CLINICAL IMPLICATIONS OF HIGH-RISK HPV DNA TEST

Because HPV DNA testing is more sensitive than cervical cytology in detecting CIN 2 and CIN 3/CIS, the clinical implications are:

- 40–60% of ASC-US Paps will be positive for high-risk HPV.
- Adding HPV tests raises the Pap sensitivity from 51 to 96%.
- 3–10% of high-risk HPV DNA-positive women will develop HSIL (CIN 2, 3/CIS).

- Only 0.7% of high-risk HPV DNA-negative women will develop HSIL (CIN 2, 3/CIS).
- Women with persistent infections with high-risk virus are at a greater risk for HSIL (CIN 2, 3/CIS) and squamous cancer compared with women who have transient infections.
- Women with an abnormal Pap test and a positive high-risk HPV test are at a higher risk (6–7% or greater) of developing cervical cancer if left untreated.
- Women with normal Pap test results and negative for high-risk HPV are at a very low risk (0.2%) for developing cervical cancer.
- HPV testing should not be performed in women with LSIL, atypical squamous cells of undetermined significance, or atypical glandular cells (AGC). In the ASC-US-LSIL Triage study, 83% of LSIL and 71% of ASC cannot exclude HSIL cases were positive for high-risk HPV. The majority of AGC were proven to be SIL on follow-up, and the HPV test may help in the initial management of these cases. The detection of HPV in women referred for AGC is shown to be 28%.

10

Atypical Squamous Cells

INTRODUCTION

Epithelial cell abnormality of squamous cell type, subcategorized as:

- Atypical squamous cells of undetermined significance (ASC-US).
- Atypical squamous cells cannot exclude high-grade squamous intra-epithelial lesion (ASC-H).

BASIC INFORMATION REGARDING ASC

- ASC is the most common abnormal cervical cytological diagnosis accounting for approx 2 million Pap test diagnoses.
- ASC is not highly reproducible.
- In general, ASC should comprise 5% or less of Pap test results. In high-risk clinics, the ASC rate should not exceed two to three times the squamous intra-epithelial lesion (SIL) rate. Thus, the ASC/SIL ratio is a better indicator of ASC rate.
- Median ASC/SIL ratio in the United States is 2.0. The ASC/SIL ratio for a conventional smear is 1.4, and for a liquid-based preparations (LBP) is 1.3.

ASC-US

- Definition: Cytological changes suggestive of SIL, but are quantitatively or qualitatively insufficient for a definitive interpretation. The category includes:
  - A minority of cases formally classified as ASC-US, favor reactive.
  - Most cases formally classified as ASC-US, not otherwise specified or ASC-US, favor SIL.
- ASC-US represents 90–95% of ASC Pap test diagnoses.
- Subsequent high-grade squamous intra-epithelial lesions (HSIL) are found in 5–17% of cases.
- Management strategies include repeat Pap test, reflex human papillomavirus (HPV) test, and direct colposcopy.

Morphological Features of ASC-US (Figs. 10.1–10.3)

- Cell type: superficial and intermediate squamous cells.
- Nuclei: round, relatively smooth contour, two and a half to three times the size of an intermediate cell, slightly hyperchromatic.
- Cytoplasm: may show a vague cytoplasmic cavitation.
- Nuclear-to-cytoplasmic (n:c) ratio: slight increase.
- These subtle features of ASC-US are better appreciated on LBP.

From: *Fundamentals of Pap Test Cytology*
By: R. S. Hoda and S. A. Hoda © Humana Press Inc., Totowa, NJ

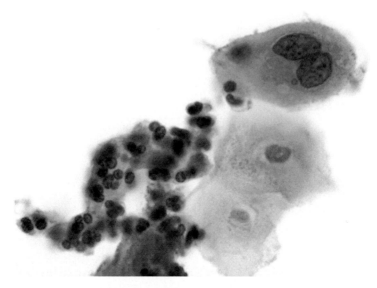

Fig. 10.1. Atypical squamous cells of undetermined significance, not otherwise specified. Enlarged, hyperchromatic, binucleated cell in an inflammatory background (ThinPrep; Papanicolaou stain).

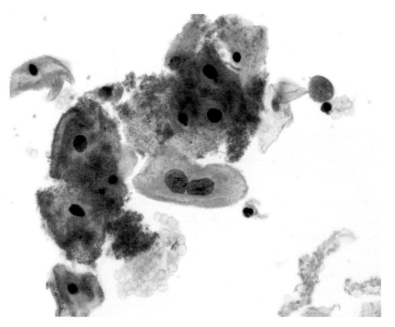

Fig. 10.2. Atypical squamous cells of undetermined significance, not otherwise specified. Single, binucleated cell with slight nuclear enlargement and irregularity (ThinPrep; Papanicolaou stain).

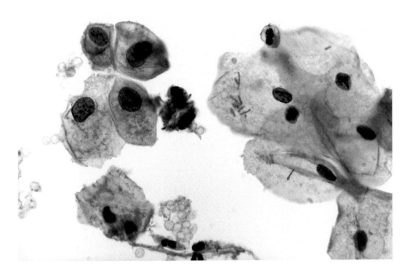

Fig. 10.3. Atypical squamous cells of undetermined significance, not otherwise specified. Cells with slight nuclear enlargement and hyperchromasia (ThinPrep; Papanicolaou stain).

ASC-US Variants

- Equivocal changes of HPV.
- Atypical repair.
- Atypical parakeratosis.
- Atypical atrophy.

Cytological Features of ASC-US With Equivocal Changes of HPV (Figs. 10.4 and 10.5)

- Ill-defined perinuclear halos (koilocytotes) with or without nuclear abnormalities.
- Nuclei are mostly eccentric, bi-, or multinucleated with smudged dark chromatin or pyknosis.

Cytological Features of ASC-US, Atypical Repair (Figs. 10.6 and 10.7)

- Atypia exceeds typical repair.
- Cellular crowding and overlap.
- Slightly dyscohesive, single cells.
- Nuclei: piling, loss of polarity, anisonucleosis, irregular nuclear contour, uneven dark chromatin, prominent single or multiple nucleoli.
- Relatively increased n:c ratio.
- Mitosis present.
- Inflammatory background, no tumor diathesis.
- Differential diagnosis includes invasive cancer.

Cytological Features of ASC-US, Atypical Parakeratosis (Figs. 10.8 and 10.9)

- Sheets, three-dimensional clusters, or single, miniature, mature squamous cells.
- Irregular cell shapes with spindle cell forms.

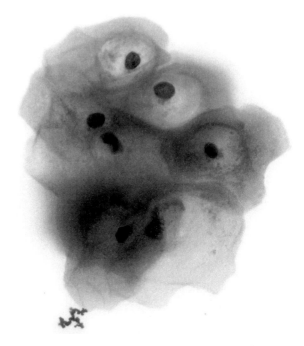

Fig. 10.4. Atypical squamous cells of undetermined significance, suggestive of human papillomavirus effect. Note suggestion of koilocytotic halo (SurePath; Papanicolaou stain).

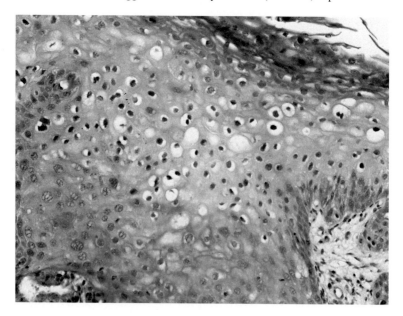

Fig. 10.5. Condyloma (human papillomavirus effect) of cervix. Same case as in Fig. 10.4 (H&E stain).

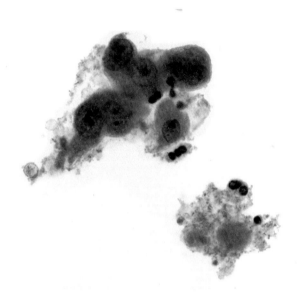

Fig. 10.6. Atypical squamous cells of undetermined significance, atypical repair. Enlarged atypical nuclei with relatively high nuclear-to-cytoplasmic ratio (ThinPrep; Papanicolaou stain).

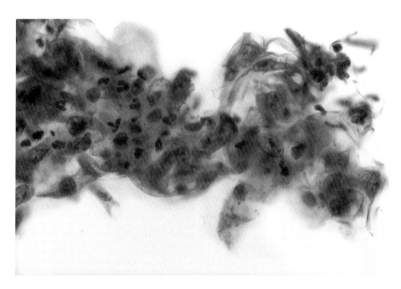

Fig. 10.7. Atypical squamous cells of undetermined significance, atypical repair. Cells with "streaming" effect and inflammation characteristic of repair. However, the nuclear atypia and loss of polarity make it atypical (ThinPrep; Papanicolaou stain).

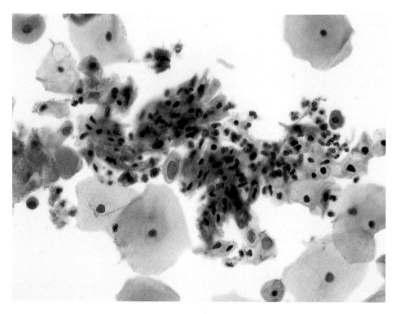

Fig. 10.8. Atypical squamous cells of undetermined significance, atypical parakeratosis. Miniature squamous cells with slightly enlarged pleomorphic nuclei (conventional smear; Papanicolaou stain).

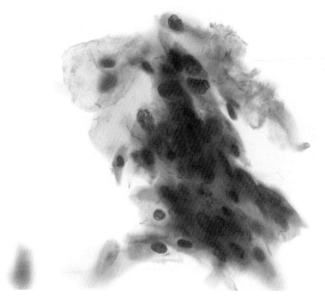

Fig. 10.9. Atypical squamous cells of undetermined significance, atypical parakeratosis. Nuclei are hyperchromatic and irregular (ThinPrep; Papanicolaou stain).

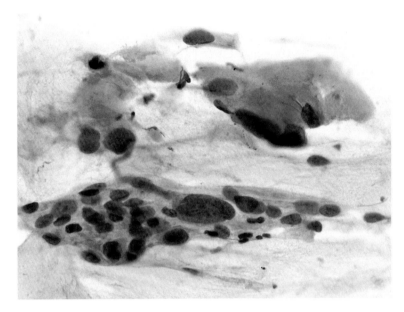

Fig. 10.10. Atypical squamous cells of undetermined significance, atypical atrophy. This 80-year-old patient showed nuclear enlargement, hyperchromasia, and pleomorphism (conventional smear; Papanicolaou stain).

- Spindled, elongated, hyperchromatic or pyknotic nuclei with tapered ends.
- Slightly high n:c ratio.
- Deeply eosinophilic cytoplasm.
- On liquid-based cytology atypical parakeratosis usually forms plaques.

MIMICS OF ATYPICAL PARAKERATOSIS

- Degenerative changes.
- Marked atrophy.

Cytological Features of ASC-US, Atypical Atrophy (Figs. 10.10 and 10.11)

- Nuclear enlargement, at least greater than two times normal parabasal cells.
- Significant hyperchromasia.
- Irregular nuclear contours or chromatin distribution.
- Nuclear pleomorphism.

Benign Mimics of ASC-US

- Inflammation-associated changes (Fig. 10.12).
- Therapy changes of radiation (Fig. 10.13).
- Glycogenated intermediate cells (Fig. 10.14).
- Parakeratosis.
- Atrophy.
- Decidual cells.
- Folic acid deficiency.

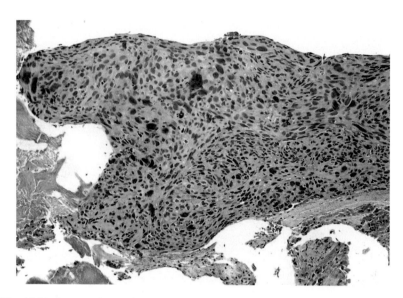

Fig. 10.11. Same patient as in Fig. 10.10. Showed a high-grade squamous intra-epithelial lesion in the setting of atrophy on subsequent cervix biopsy (H&E stain).

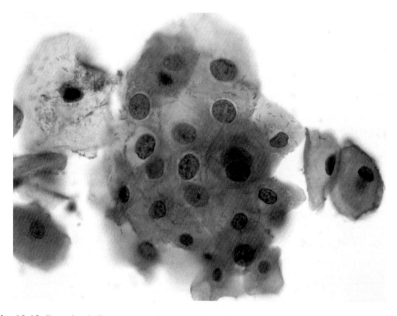

Fig. 10.12. Reactive inflammatory changes with slight nuclear enlargement and perinuclear halo may mimic low-grade squamous intra-epithelial lesion. Note the uniform, normochromic nuclei (ThinPrep; Papanicolaou stain).

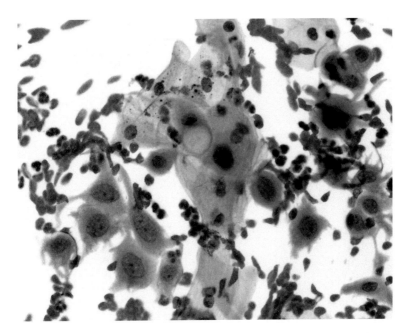

Fig. 10.13. Radiation effect with nuclear enlargement may mimic low-grade squamous intra-epithelial lesion (conventional smear; Papanicolaou stain).

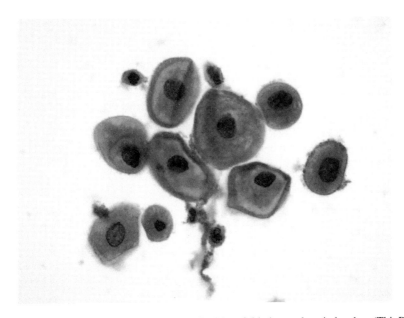

Fig. 10.14. Glycogenated intermediate cells. Note folded cytoplasmic borders (ThinPrep; Papanicolaou stain).

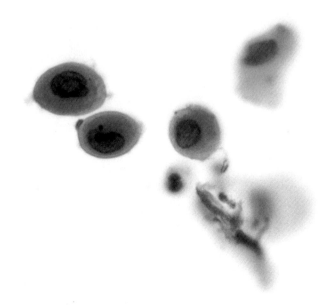

Fig. 10.15. Atypical squamous cells cannot exclude HSIL. Single metaplastic-type cells with nuclear hyperchromasia, irregularity, and a slight increase in the nuclear-to-cytoplasmic ratio (ThinPrep; Papanicolaou stain).

- Cytotrophoblasts.
- Air-drying artifact.

ASC-H

- Definition: Cytological changes suggestive of HSIL but lack criteria for a definitive interpretation. The association with underlying cervical intra-epithelial neoplasia 2 and 3 for ASC-H is lower than for HSIL, but sufficiently higher than for ASC-US to warrant consideration of different management recommendations.
- ASC-H represents 5–10% of all Pap tests diagnoses.
- Subsequent HSIL is seen in 30–40% of cases.
- Management of ASC-H is colposcopy.

Cytological Features of ASC-H (Figs. 10.15–10.19)

- Few abnormal cells.
- Dispersed singly, loosely cohesive groups in an immature cell pattern, hyperchromati-crowded group.
- Cell size is of metaplastic cells with variation in size and shape.
- Nuclei: one and a half to two times normal metaplastic cells or three times intermediate cell nuclei, hyperchromasia, slight membrane irregularity, variation in size and shape, small nucleoli may be present.
- Cytoplasm: metaplastic to lacy with distinct outlines.
- Increased n:c ratio.
- All the features are better appreciated on LBP.

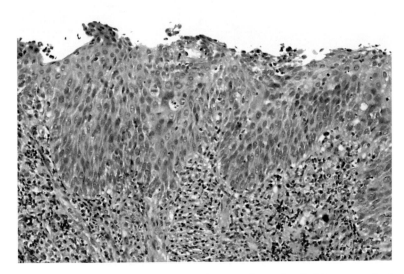

Fig. 10.16. Cervical intra-epithelial neoplasia II (moderate dysplasia) was seen in the case in Fig. 10.15 on subsequent cervix biopsy (H&E stain).

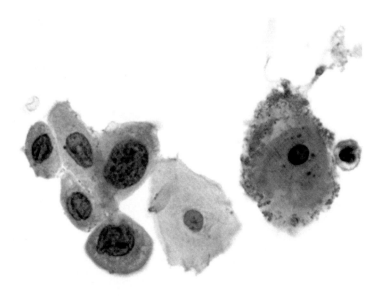

Fig. 10.17. Atypical squamous cells cannot exclude HSIL. The only atypical cell seen on the Pap test in this case (ThinPrep; Papanicolaou stain).

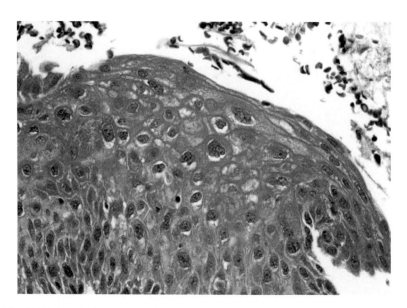

Fig. 10.18. Cervical intra-epithelial neoplasia II (moderate dysplasia) was seen in the case in Fig. 10.17 on subsequent cervix biopsy (H&E stain).

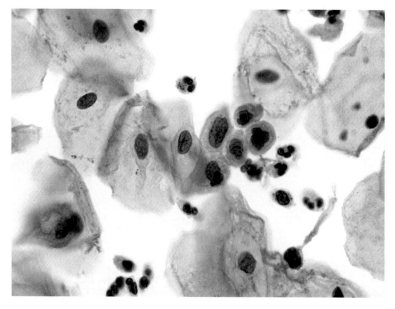

Fig. 10.19. Atypical squamous cells cannot exclude HSIL. A group of small atypical cells with irregular nuclear membranes and hyperchromasia (SurePath; Papanicolaou stain).

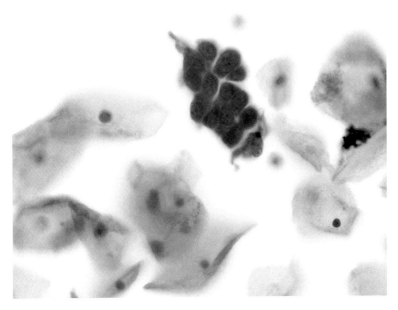

Fig. 10.20. Reactive endocervical cells may mimic atypical squamous cells cannot exclude HSIL. Note uniformity of nuclei and small nucleoli (SurePath; Papanicolaou stain).

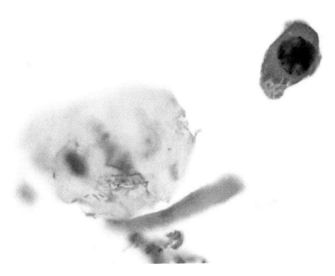

Fig. 10.21. Degenerated endocervical cells may mimic atypical squamous cells cannot exclude HSIL. Note poorly preserved nuclei with smudged chromatin (ThinPrep; Papanicolaou stain).

Benign Mimics of ASC-H

- Reactive endocervical cells (Fig. 10.20).
- Nuclear degeneration (Fig. 10.21).
- Squamous metaplasia.
- Repair.
- Atrophy.
- Degenerated endometrial cells.
- Intrauterine device-associated cells.
- Histiocytes.
- Pregnancy-associated changes.
- Microglandular hyperplasia.

MANAGEMENT OF ASC

Please *see* Chapter 19.

11
Low-Grade Squamous Intra-Epithelial Lesion

EPITHELIAL CELL ABNORMALITY OF SQUAMOUS CELL TYPE

- Low-grade squamous intra-epithelial lesion (LSIL) encompasses both human papillomavirus (HPV) effects and mild dysplasia (cervical intra-epithelial neoplasia [CIN] 1).
- Approximately 80% of high-risk HPV (+) women have CIN 1 on subsequent biopsy.
- Approximately 9–16% have high-grade squamous intra-epithelial lesion 2–3 on subsequent biopsy.
- Spontaneous regression is seen in approx 57% of CIN 1 cases.
- Progression to CIN 2, 3 is seen in 11% of CIN 1 cases.
- Squamous-cell carcinoma may develop in 0.3% of women with CIN 1.
- As there is no reliable indicator of which women with CIN 1 will progress to a higher grade lesion, some form of surveillance is indicated.

CYTOLOGICAL FEATURES OF LSIL WITH HPV EFFECT (FIGS. 11.1–11.3)

- Nuclei are variable compared with normal-intermediate cell nuclei.
- May be enlarged, equal to normal intermediate cell nucleus, or pyknotic.
- Chromatin is smudged.
- Nuclear membrane wrinkling (raisinoid).
- Mature cytoplasm.
- Koilocytes appear as distinct cave-like cytoplasmic vacuoles—perinuclear halo.
- Sharp, dense periphery and condensed cytoplasm.

CYTOMORPHOLOGY OF LSIL, MILD DYSPLASIA (FIGS. 11.4 AND 11.5)

- Mature squamous cells, superficial or intermediate cell type.
- Single or in sheets.
- Nuclei is more than four to six times a normal intermediate cell nucleus.
- Hyperchromatic with finely granular chromatin.
- Irregular nuclear membrane.
- Nucleoli rare and inconspicuous.
- Nuclear-to-cytoplasmic ratio is relatively high.
- Better detection of LSIL on liquid-based preparations has reduced atypical squamous cell: squamous intra-epithelial lesion ratio (Table 1).

From: *Fundamentals of Pap Test Cytology*
By: R. S. Hoda and S. A. Hoda © Humana Press Inc., Totowa, NJ

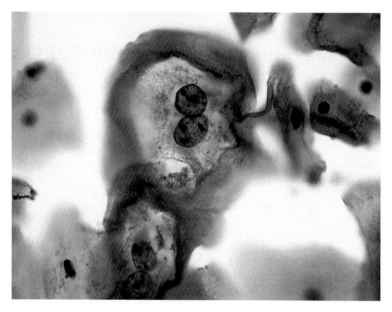

Fig. 11.1. Low-grade squamous intra-epithelial lesion-human papillomavirus. Note the prominent, optically clear perinuclear halo (koilocytes) (SurePath; Papanicolaou stain).

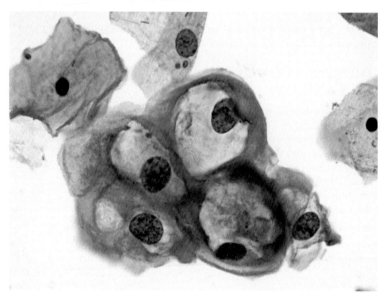

Fig. 11.2. Low-grade squamous intra-epithelial lesion-human papillomavirus (ThinPrep; Papanicolaou stain).

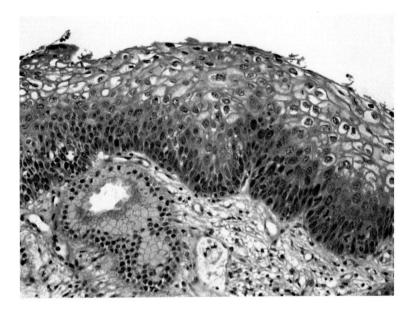

Fig. 11.3. Condyloma (H&E stain).

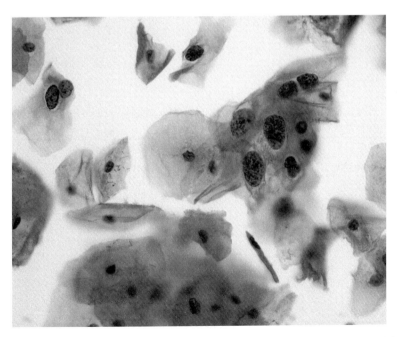

Fig. 11.4. Low-grade squamous intra-epithelial lesion, mild dysplasia (cervical intra-epithelial neoplasia I) (SurePath; Papanicolaou stain).

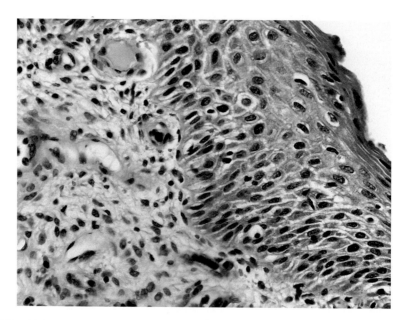

Fig. 11.5. Low-grade squamous intra-epithelial lesion (mild dysplasia, cervical intra-epithelial neoplasia 1) (H&E stain).

Table 1
Low-Grade Squamous Intra-Epithelial Lesion vs High-Grade Squamous Intra-Epithelial Lesion, Cytological Features

Abnormality	LSIL	HSIL
Cell arrangement	Single/sheet	Single/sheet/syncytial
Cell type	Superficial and intermediate	Metaplastic
Nucleus	Enlarged	Small to enlarged
Chromatin	Granular[a]	Coarsely granular
Nuclear membrane	Irregular +/–	Irregular++, Indentation, grooves
Nucleolus	–	+/–
Binucleation	++	–
Mitosis	Rare	Frequent
Cytoplasm	Mature	Metaplastic or lacy
Koilocytes	++ in HPV	–
N:c ratio	Increased +	Increased ++

[a]Opaque or smudged in HPV.

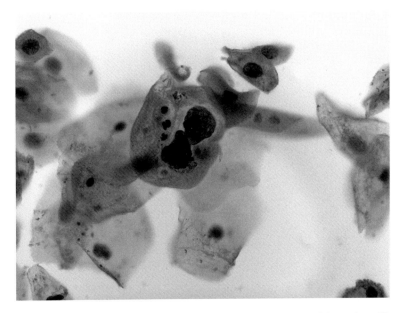

Fig. 11.6. Low-grade squamous intra-epithelial lesion-human papillomavirus. Note the raisin-like nuclei (ThinPrep; Papanicolaou stain).

MIMICS OF LSIL

The cytological features of bi- or multinucleation and nuclear enlargement seen in LSIL (Figs. 11.6 and 11.7) may be mimicked by:

- Glycogenated intermediate (navicular) cells (Fig. 11.8).
- Reactive inflammatory changes (Fig. 11.9).
- Air-drying.
- Degenerated cells.
- Folic acid deficiency.
- Repair including treatment effects of radiation.
- Atrophy.

FALSE-NEGATIVE LSIL

- False-negative rate for LSIL is less than that for high-grade squamous intra-epithelial lesion.
- Missed LSIL cases have fewer abnormal cells with a median number less than 50.
- Cases with 101–250 LSIL cells are easily detected.

MANAGEMENT GUIDELINES FOR LSIL

Please *see* Chapter 19.

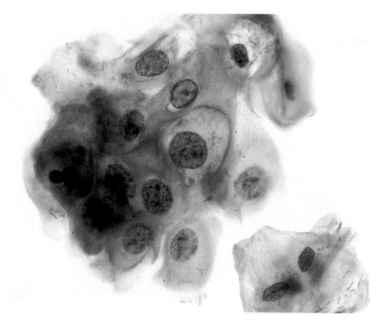

Fig. 11.7. Low-grade squamous intra-epithelial lesion, human papillomavirus, and mild dyplasia (ThinPrep; Papanicolaou stain).

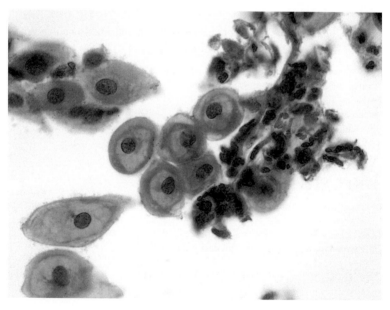

Fig. 11.8. Glycogenated intermediate cells may mimic koilocytes. The nuclei, however, are uniform (ThinPrep; Papanicolaou stain).

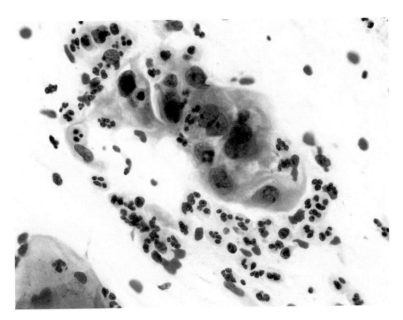

Fig. 11.9. Reactive inflammatory changes with bi- or multinucleation may mimic low-grade squamous intra-epithelial lesion. Note the presence of regular nuclei, nucleoli, and inflammation (conventional smear; Papanicolaou stain).

12

High-Grade Squamous Intra-Epithelial Lesion

EPITHELIAL CELL ABNORMALITY OF SQUAMOUS CELL TYPE

- High-grade squamous intra-epithelial lesion (HSIL) includes moderate dysplasia (cervical intra-epithelial neoplasia 2), severe dysplasia, and carcinoma *in situ* (cervical intra-epithelial neoplasia 3/carcinoma *in situ*).
- There is wide variation in the cytological appearance of HSIL.
- As the severity of dysplasia increases, the cell appears more immature. There is an increase in the nuclear size and atypia therein, a decrease in the cytoplasm, and an increase in the nuclear-to-cytoplasmic (n:c) ratio.
- High-risk HPV is found in 97% of women with HSIL.

DIAGNOSTIC CRITERIA OF HSIL (FIGS. 12.1–12.7)

- Cells appear singly, in sheets, or in syncytial fragments.
- Cells are of parabasal, basal, or metaplastic type.0
- Nuclei are three times the size of intermediate cell nuclei (same range as low-grade squamous intra-epithelial lesion). There is variation in the size and the shape of the nuclei.
- Nuclei are hyperchromatic with coarse, evenly distributed chromatin.
- Nuclear membrane is markedly irregular.
- Nucleoli may be present.
- Cytoplasm is "immature," dense or lacy, and delicate.
- Cytoplasm is eosinophilic/orangeophilic in keratinizing dysplasia.
- High n:c.
- Hyperchromatic crowded groups are mostly seen in carcinoma *in situ*.
- On liquid-based preparations, nuclear abnormalities are more pronounced because of the absence of obscuring features, single cells are more common, and streaking of abnormal cells is not seen because of specimen processing.

HSIL INVOLVING ENDOCERVICAL GLANDS (FIGS. 12.5 AND 12.7)

- Hyperchromatic-crowded groups or large syncytial aggregates with ill-defined cell borders.
- Cells within the cluster show overlapping loss of polarity.
- Peripheral flattening of cells.
- Nucleoli are not seen.

From: *Fundamentals of Pap Test Cytology*
By: R. S. Hoda and S. A. Hoda © Humana Press Inc., Totowa, NJ

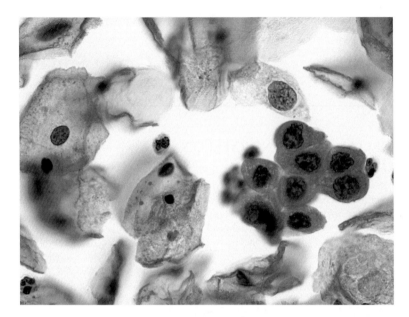

Fig. 12.1. Small group of high-grade squamous intra-epithelial lesions. Nuclei are hyperchromatic and irregular (SurePath; Papanicolaou stain).

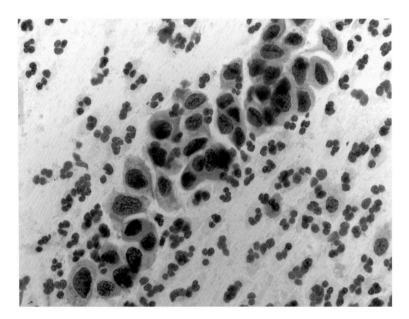

Fig. 12.2. Loose sheet of high-grade squamous intra-epithelial lesions (conventional smear; Papanicolaou stain).

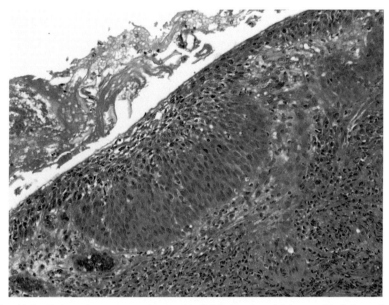

Fig. 12.3. High-grade squamous intra-epithelial lesion (cervial intra-epithelial neoplasia 3, severe dysplasia, carcinoma *in situ*) in cervical biopsy from the same case as in Fig. 12.2 (H&E stain).

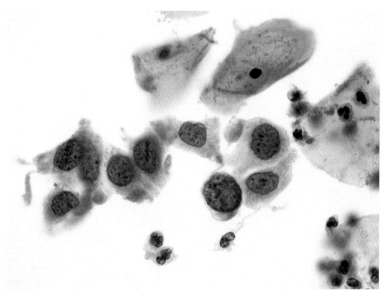

Fig. 12.4. High-grade squamous intra-epithelial lesion. Note the metaplastic-type cells with coarse chromatin, nuclear membrane irregularity, and high nuclear-to-cytoplasmic ratio (ThinPrep; Papanicolaou stain).

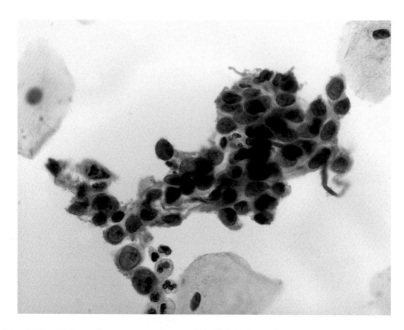

Fig. 12.5. High-grade squamous intra-epithelial lesion with endocervical gland involvement. Note the hyperchromatic irregular nuclei with peripheral flattening (ThinPrep; Papanicolaou stain).

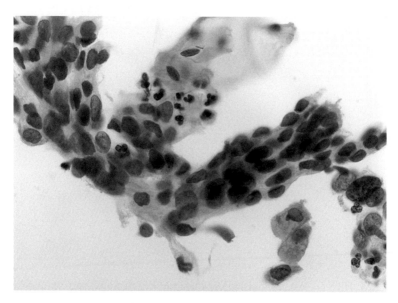

Fig. 12.6. High-grade squamous intra-epithelial lesion (HSIL) syncytia. Irregularly arranged HSIL cells (ThinPrep; Papanicolaou stain).

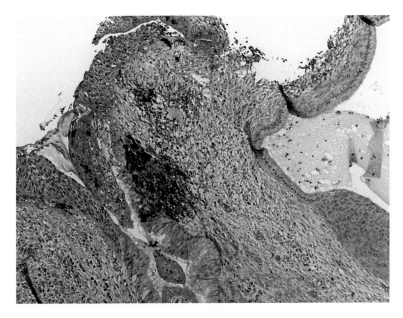

Fig. 12.7. High-grade squamous intra-epithelial lesion with endocervical gland involvement in cervical biopsy from same case as in Fig. 12.5 (H&E stain).

BENIGN MIMICS OF HSIL

- Squamous metaplasia (Fig. 12.8).
- Sheets of basal/parabasal cells in atrophy (Fig. 12.9).
- Histiocytes (Fig. 12.10).
- Microglandular hyperplasia, metaplastic type (Fig. 12.11).
- Pseudokeratinized cells in atrophy.
- Follicular cervicitis.
- Reserve cell hyperplasia.
- Endometrial cells.
- Endocervical cells.
- Transitional metaplasia.
- Reserve cells.
- Intrauterine contraceptive device.
- Overstained cells.
  - HSIL shows large nuclear size, coarseness of nuclear chromatin, a nuclear groove, and abnormalities of nuclear contour. These benign entities show homogenously fine chromatin and smooth nuclear contours.

NEOPLASTIC DIFFERENTIAL DIAGNOSIS OF HSIL

- **Adenocarcinoma *in situ* (Fig. 12.12):** Adenocarcinoma *in situ* characteristically shows peripheral nuclear palisading *"feathering,"* nucleoli, and apoptosis.
- **Squamous-cell carcinoma, large-cell nonkeratinizing:** This tumor is distinguished from HSIL by the presence of macronucleoli and necrotic tumor diathesis.

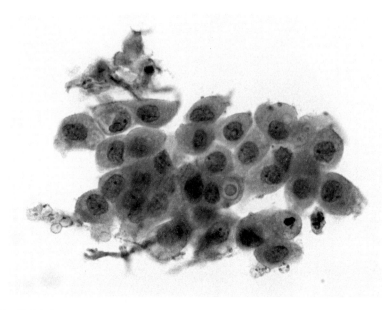

Fig. 12.8. Mature squamous metaplasia may mimic high-grade squamous intra-epithelial lesion. Nuclei are pale (ThinPrep; Papanicolaou stain).

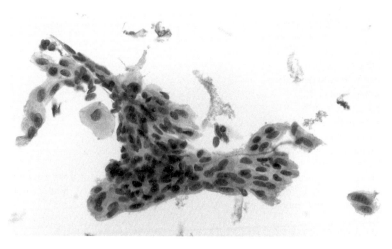

Fig. 12.9. Parabasal cells in atrophy may mimic syncytia of high-grade squamous intra-epithelial lesion. Note the pale, uniform nuclei (ThinPrep; Papanicolaou stain).

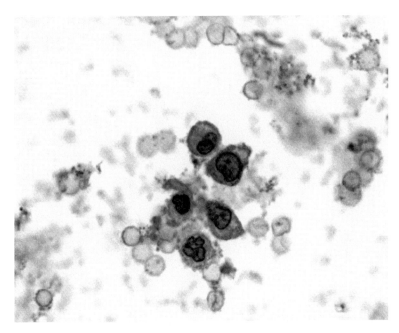

Fig. 12.10. Histiocytes with a small size and a relatively high nuclear-to-cytoplasmic ratio may mimic high-grade squamous intra-epithelial lesion. Note reniform pale nuclei (conventional smear; Papanicolaou stain).

- **Squamous-cell carcinoma, keratinizing:** Keratinizing squamous carcinoma shows more cellular and nuclear pleomorphism and tumor diathesis.
- **Small-cell carcinoma:** Small-cell carcinoma shows aggregates of small, round, blue cells with nuclear molding, crush artifact, and individual tumor cell necrosis (apoptosis).

KERATINIZING HSIL (FIGS. 12.13 AND 12.14)

- High cellularity.
- Atypical cells occur singly or in sheets.
- Pleomorphic cell shapes with spindle and elongated and tadpole forms.
- Nuclei are dark with size and shape variation, and the membrane is irregular.
- Cytoplasm is dense and orangeophilic.
- High n:c.
- Mitoses may be present.
- Tumor diathesis is absent.
- Differential diagnosis includes keratinizing squamous-cell carcinoma, atrophic vaginitis with pseudokeratinized cells, and pseudoparakeratosis (Fig. 12.15).

MANAGEMENT GUIDELINES ON HSIL

Please *see* Chapter 19.

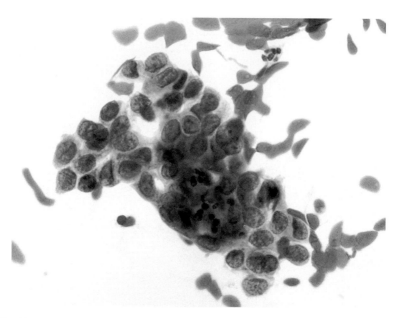

Fig. 12.11. Microglandular hyperplasia, metaplastic type may mimic high-grade squamous intra-epithelial lesion (HSIL). Nuclear features of HSIL are not seen (conventional smear; Papanicolaou stain).

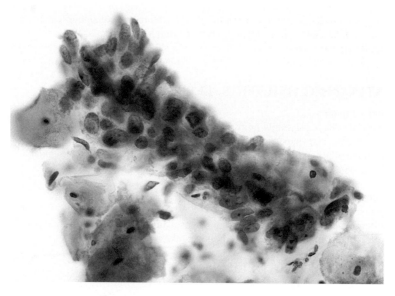

Fig. 12.12. Adenocarcinoma *in situ* may be mistaken for high-grade squamous intra-epithelial lesion with endocervical gland involvement. Note "feathering" (ThinPrep, Papanicolaou stain).

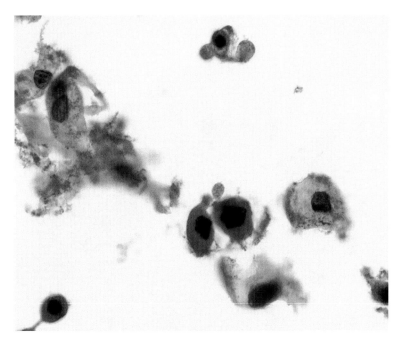

Fig. 12.13. Keratinizing dysplasia. Orangeophilic cytoplasm with rigid contours and opaque nucleus (ThinPrep; Papanicolaou stain).

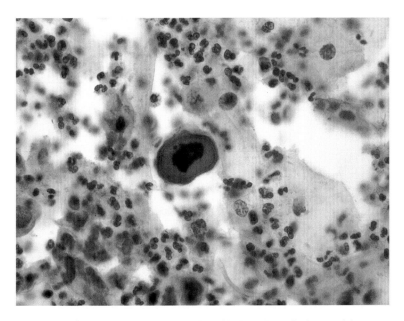

Fig. 12.14. Keratinizing dysplasia (ThinPrep; Papanicolaou stain).

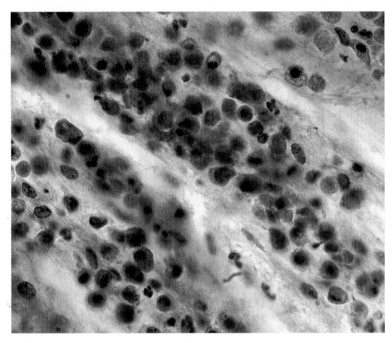

Fig. 12.15. Pseudoparakeratosis may mimic keratinizing dysplasia. Note the lack of nuclear details (conventional smear; Papanicolaou stain).

13

Invasive Squamous Carcinoma

EPITHELIAL CELL ABNORMALITY

Squamous-Cell Carcinoma of the Cervix, Basics

- Most common malignant tumor of the cervix.
- Usually occurs between 45–55 years of age.

TYPES OF INVASIVE CARCINOMA (TABLES 1 AND 2)

- Well-differentiated keratinizing carcinoma.
- Large-cell nonkeratinizing carcinoma.
- Small-cell carcinoma.

PROGNOSTIC FACTORS

- Depth of invasion.
- Lymphovascular invasion.
- Keratin formation and tumor grade do not appear to influence prognosis.

DEFINITION OF MICROINVASIVE CARCINOMA OF THE CERVIX

Defined as a carcinoma, which on histological sections invades the underlying stroma for a distance of 5 mm or less, and has a horizontal spread of 7 mm or less.

A reliable cytological diagnosis of microinvasive carcinoma cannot be made.

Cytological Features of Microinvasive Carcinoma

- Cells resemble those of high-grade squamous intra-epithelial lesion (HSIL) or invasive carcinoma.
- Large number of atypical cells.
- Cells may be present in syncytial arrangement.
- Presence of nucleoli favors microinvasion.
- Eosinophilic cytoplasm is a feature to look for.
- Background may be inflammatory.

CYTOLOGICAL FEATURES OF KERATINIZING CARCINOMA (FIGS. 13.1–13.5)

- Usually originate in the squamous epithelium of the ectocervix.
- May form a protruding tumor.

From: *Fundamentals of Pap Test Cytology*
By: R. S. Hoda and S. A. Hoda © Humana Press Inc., Totowa, NJ

Table 1
Cytological Features of Various Types of Squamous Neoplasia

Abnormality	Carcinoma *in situ*	Microinvasive[a]	Invasive carcinoma
Cell shape	Round to ovoid	Tapered (fiber cells)	Bizarre
Nucleus	Small	Enlarged +	Enlarged ++
Chromatin	Irregular –	Irregular +	Irregular ++
Nucleoli	+/–	+	Prominent
Diathesis	–	+/–	++

[a]*See* p. 113.
–, absent; +, present; ++, common.

Table 2
Cytological Features of Various Types of Squamous Carcinoma

Features	Keratinizing	Nonkeratinizing	Small cell
Single cells	++	+	+
Cell clusters	+	++	++
Cell Shape	Bizarre/spindle	Round/polygonal	Ovoid
Cell variance	Pleomorphic	Variable	Uniform
Cytoplasm	Orangeophilic	Cyanophilic	Basophilic
Nucleolus	+/–	++	+
Diathesis	+/–	++	+
N:c	Variable	High	High

N:c, nuclear-to-cytoplasmic ratio.
–, absent; +, present; ++, common.

- Pleomorphic caudate or tadpole-shaped cells and "fiber" cells (Figs. 13.3 and 13.4).
- Size of cells is variable.
- Nuclei are hyperchromatic, opaque, or pyknotic with coarse irregular chromatin and parachromatin clearing.
- Nucleoli are variable.
- Cytoplasm is dense and orangeophilic with distinct and rigid cell borders.
- Tumor diathesis is generally present.
- On liquid-based preparations (LBP) orangeophilia is more pronounced.

Differential Diagnosis of Keratinizing Cells

- Hyperkeratosis.
- Parakeratosis.
- Atypical parakeratosis.
- Human papillomavirus-associated cellular changes.
- Pseudoparakeratosis in menopause.
- Reactive pearl formation.
- Keratinizing dysplasia.
  - *Note:* keratinizing squamous-cell carcinoma is distinguished from these entities by the presence of cellular pleomorphism and tumor diathesis. A previous history of an abnormal Pap test may be present in carcinoma.

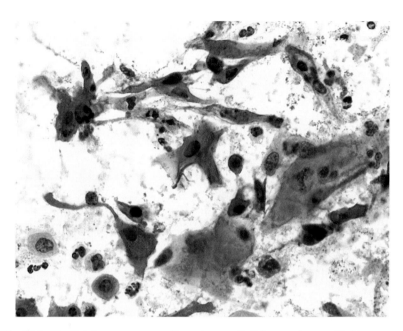

Fig. 13.1. Keratinizing squamous-cell carcinoma. Cellular specimen with bizarre opaque nuclei and orangeophilic cytoplasm. Compare with Fig. 13.2 (conventional smear; Papanicolaou stain).

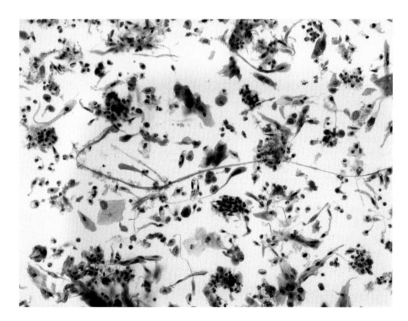

Fig. 13.2. Keratinizing squamous-cell carcinoma. Compare with Fig. 13.1 (SurePath; Papanicolaou stain).

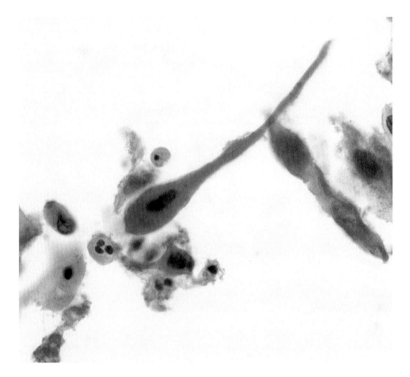

Fig. 13.3. "Tadpole" or "caudate" cell in keratinizing squamous-cell carcinoma (ThinPrep; Papanicolaou stain).

LARGE CELL NONKERATINIZING CARCINOMA (FIGS. 13.6 AND 13.7)

- Arises from the transformation zone.
- Less cellular pleomorphism than keratinizing carcinoma.
- Sheets, thick clusters, syncytial fragments, and single cells.
- Cells of variable size.
- Resembles HSIL, plus coarser chromatin and prominent nucleoli.
- Clearing of parachromatin is usually a feature.
- Cytoplasm may be poorly preserved.
- Mitoses may be present.
- Necrotic diathesis seen.
- On LBP the diathesis is clumped and clings to tumor cells, called clinging diathesis. It does not obscure cell detail.

Differential Diagnosis of Nonkeratinizing Squamous Carcinoma (Fig. 13.8)

- Adenocarcinoma (Table 3).
- Metastatic tumor.

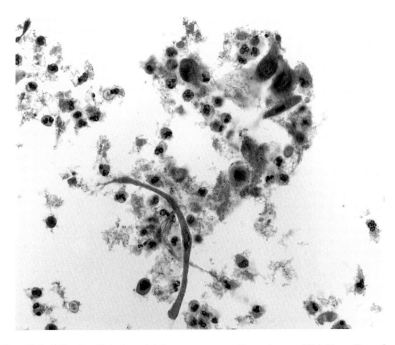

Fig. 13.4. "Fiber" cell in keratinizing squamous-cell carcinoma (ThinPrep; Papanicolaou stain).

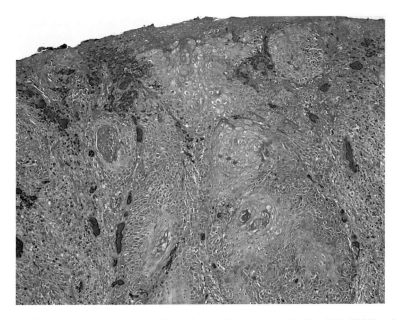

Fig. 13.5. Keratinizing squamous-cell carcinoma. Same case as in Fig. 13.1 (H&E stain).

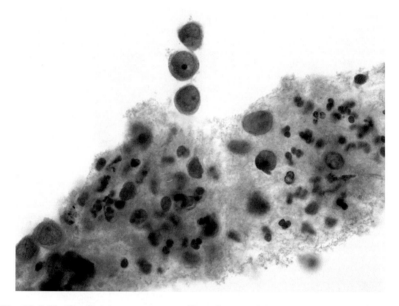

Fig. 13.6. Nonkeratinizing squamous-cell carcinoma with clinging tumor diathesis. Cells are round with hyperchromatic centrally placed nuclei and dense cytoplasm (ThinPrep; Papanicolaou stain).

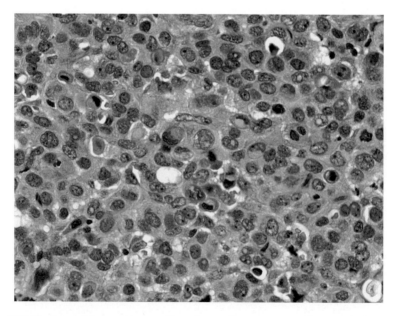

Fig. 13.7. Nonkeratinizing squamous-cell carcinoma. Same case as in Fig. 13.16 (H&E stain).

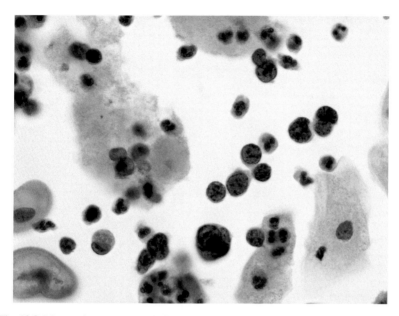

Fig. 13.8. Metastatic mammary lobular carcinoma on a Pap test. Note the linear arrangement of small round cells with eccentric irregular nuclei and nucleoli. Cytoplasm is delicate compared with nonkeratinizing squamous-cell carcinoma seen in Fig. 13.6 (ThinPrep; Papanicolaou stain).

Table 3
Squamous vs Adenocarcinoma on Pap Smears

Squamous carcinoma	Adenocarcinoma
Nucleus opaque	Vesicular
Nucleoli may be present	Nucleoli present
Keratin in cytoplasm	Vacuoles in cytoplasm
intracytoplasmic neutrophils-	Intracytoplasmic neutrophils++
"Pearl" formation	Duct formation
"Tadpole" cells	Papillae may be present
Flattened cell aggregates	Three-dimensional cell aggregates
Crisper cell borders	Less crisp borders
Cells in isolation	Cells in aggregates
Necrotic diathesis	Watery diathesis

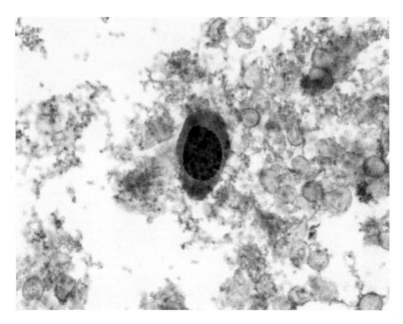

Fig. 13.9. Squamous-cell carcinoma in atrophy with granular diathesis may mimic "blue blobs." Note nuclear features (ThinPrep; Papanicolaou stain).

- Atrophy.
- Repair.
- Pemphigus.
- Pollen.

DIFFERENTIAL DIAGNOSIS OF SPINDLY CELLS ON A PAP TEST

- Fibroblasts.
- Smooth muscle cells.
- Endometrial stromal cells.
- Atrophy.
- Contaminant.
- Sarcoma.

BACKGROUND ON LBP, ATROPHIC VAGINITIS VS SQUAMOUS CARCINOMA (FIGS. 13.9–13.11)

- Seen in both atrophic vaginitis and squamous-cell carcinoma.
  - Heavy granular material.
  - Aacute inflammatory cells.
  - Apoptosis.
  - Red blood cells, fresh and crenated.

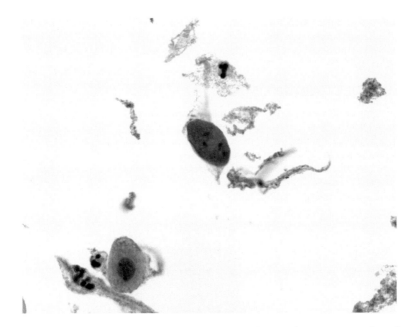

Fig. 13.10. "Blue blob" in atrophic vaginitis may be mistaken for squamous-cell carcinoma. Nuclear details and cytoplasm, as seen in Fig. 13.9, are lacking (ThinPrep; Papanicolaou stain).

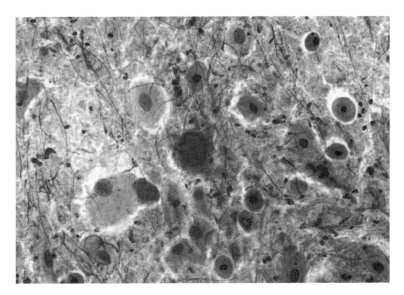

Fig. 13.11. Typical appearance of atrophic vaginitis with "blue blobs" (conventional smear; Papanicolaou stain).

- Seen in squamous carcinoma.
  - Malignant squamous cells.
- Occasionally "blue blobs" seen in atrophy may mimic squamous carcinoma cells and vice versa.

SMALL-CELL CARCINOMA

- This type of tumor originates in the endocervical canal.
- Constitutes 2–5% of cervical carcinoma.
- Morphological features similar to small-cell carcinoma of the lung.
- Appear as single cells or in syncytial fragments.
- Nuclei are small, round, dense, and hyperchromatic with occasional molding.
- Cytoplasm is scant and may be vacuolated.
- Nuclear-to-cytoplasmic ratio is high.
- Mitoses are usually seen.
- Some tumors are positive for neuroendocrine markers.

Differential Diagnosis of Small-Cell Carcinoma

- Reserve cell hyperplasia.
- Endometrial cells.
- Follicular cervicitis.
- "Bare" nuclei in atrophy.
- Small cells associated with tamoxifen therapy.
- HSIL.

14
Endocervical Lesions

EPITHELIAL CELL ABNORMALITY

Atypical Glandular Cells

In Bethesda 2001, atypical glandular cells are classified as:

- Atypical glandular cells (AGC).
  - Atypical endocervical cells (EC).
  - Atypical endometrial cells.
  - Not otherwise specified (NOS).
- AGC.
  - Atypical endocervical cells, favor neoplastic.
  - AGC favor neoplastic.
- Endocervical adenocarcinoma *in situ* (AIS).
- Adenocarcinoma.
  - Endocervical.
  - Endometrial.
  - Extrauterine.
  - NOS.

- Glandular lesions are being increasingly recognized in Pap test because of better-sampling devices, such as the endocervical brush and broom, and possibly an increase in incidence.
- Changes in AGC are more pronounced than those seen in reactive glandular cells.
- AGCs lack the diagnostic features of AIS, endocervical carcinoma, or endometrial carcinoma.
- AGCs are less common than squamous abnormalities and comprise less than 1% (mean 0.3–0.5%) of all abnormal Pap diagnoses. Therefore, cytologists have less experience in recognizing glandular lesions.
- Moreover, criteria for distinguishing between non-neoplastic reactive glandular cells from neoplastic lesions are also not well established. Approximately 30% of cases thought to be glandular are detected to be squamous in nature on subsequent biopsy.
- According to the Bethesda system, whenever possible, AGC should be characterized as:
  - AGC of endocervical or endometrial origin.
  - AGC NOS.
  - AGC favor neoplastic.
- Use of liquid-based preparations (LBP) has increased both the sensitivity and specificity in the detection of glandular lesions.

From: *Fundamentals of Pap Test Cytology*
By: R. S. Hoda and S. A. Hoda © Humana Press Inc., Totowa, NJ

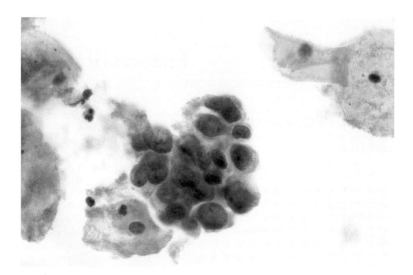

Fig. 14.1. Atypical glandular cells not otherwise specified. Three-dimensional cluster of irregular and hyperchromatic glandular cells. It cannot be determined if these cells represent endocervical vs endometrial origin (ThinPrep; Papanicolaou stain).

Cytological Features of AGC, AGC-NOS (Figs. 14.1–14.3)

- Cells occur in hyperchromatic groups, sheets, or strips.
- Nuclei are enlarged, two to three times larger than normal endocervical cell nuclei, variable.
- Slight contour irregularity and hyperchromasia.
- Nucleoli may be present.
- Cytoplasm is moderate to scant.
- Relatively high nuclear-to-cytoplasmic (n:c) ratio.
  - *Note:* It cannot be determined based on cell morphology if the cells are of endocervical or endometrial origin.

Cytological Features of AGC, Atypical EC

- Presence of some, but not all, criteria for AIS.
- Hyperchromatic-crowded group sheets or strips.
- Nuclei are enlarged (more than three times normal endocervical nuclei), minimal overlap, round to oval, mild hyperchromasia, mild loss of polarity, and small nucleoli.
- Cytoplasm is columnar and vacuolated with distinct cell borders.
- n:c high.
- Mitoses +/–.
- Appear three-dimensional (3D) on LBP; visualization of cells in the center is difficult.

Differential Diagnosis of Hyperchromatic-Crowded Groups (Fig. 14.4)

- Oversampling of endocervix.
- Tubal metaplasia.

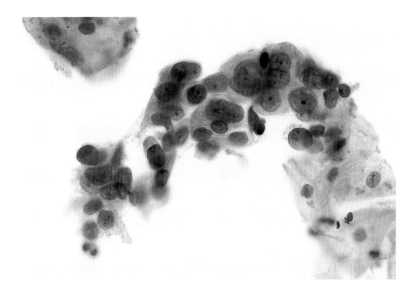

Fig. 14.2. Atypical glandular cells not otherwise specified. A strip of pleomorphic glandular cells with round-to-oval nuclei and prominent nucleoli (ThinPrep; Papanicolaou stain).

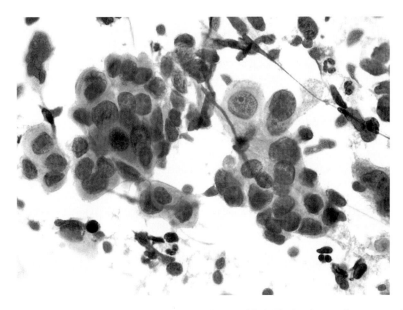

Fig. 14.3. Atypical glandular cells not otherwise specified. The background appears to have clumped debris, which may represent diathesis (conventional smear; Papanicolaou stain).

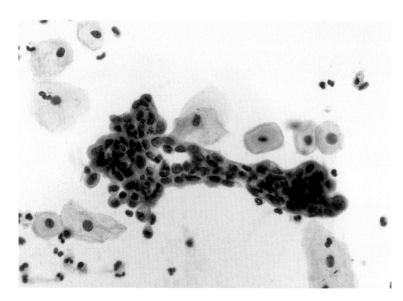

Fig. 14.4. Atypical glandular cells, favor neoplastic. Glandular cells in three-dimensional configuration with small eccentric nuclei and delicate cytoplasm. (ThinPrep; Papanicolaou stain).

- Reactive/reparative (intrauterine device, postcone, microglandular hyperplasia).
- Endometrial cells (exodus, lower uterine segment, endometriosis).
- Squamous intra-epithelial lesion (SIL).
- AIS.
- Adenocarcinoma (endocervical or endometrial).
- Nonkeratinizing squamous-cell carcinoma.
- Metastatic tumors.

Differential Diagnosis of AGC-EC

- Reactive EC are prominent with multiple nucleoli.
- Tubal metaplasia have visible cilia or terminal bar.
- Radiation change displays marked variation in cell and nuclear size.
- Intrauternine device cells have enlarged nuclei with nucleoli and vacuolated cytoplasm.
- Microglandular hyperplasia show normal endocervical cells with lumina formation.
- High-grade squamous intra-epithelial lesion (HSIL) has crowded clusters of cells, hyperchromasia, and flattening of cells toward the periphery.
- AIS.

FOLLOWUP OF AGC

- Benign: 20–40%.
- Squamous lesions: 35–80%.
- AIS: 0–11%.
- Endometrial carcinoma: 9%.

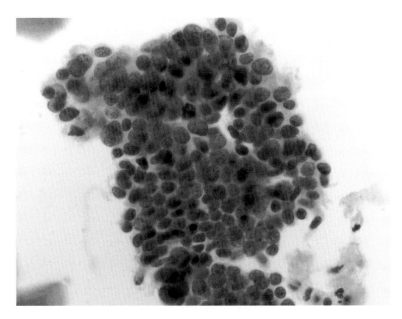

Fig. 14.5. Atypical glandular cells, atypical endocervical cells, favor neoplastic. Hyperchromatic crowded group of endocervical cells with round to oval dark nuclei. Vague peripheral palisading of nuclei is seen (ThinPrep; Papanicolaou stain).

CYTOMORPHOLOGY OF ATYPICAL ECs, FAVOR NEOPLASTIC (FIGS. 14.5 AND 14.6)

- Columnar cells in hyperchromatic crowded groups, two-dimensional (2D) sheets, strips, and rosettes.
- Pseudostratification.
- Nuclear palisading "feathering" present.
- Nuclei are enlarged, elongated, hyperchromatic, overlapping, irregular, and have a thickened contour.
- Nucleoli +/–.
- Increased n:c.
- Occasional mitoses.
  - *Note:* In postmenopausal patients, AGC is indicative of a significant pathology in 32.7% of cases.

ADEONCARCINOMA *IN SITU* (FIGS. 14.7–14.12)

AIS is a precursor lesion for endocervical adenocarcinoma and is detected several years before invasive adenocarcinoma is diagnosed. AIS is also seen in proximity to invasive cancer and both show a similar proportion of human papillomaviruses (HPV) 16 and 18. Incidence of invasive endocervical adenocarcinoma is higher than that of AIS. Sensitivity of a Pap test for AIS diagnosis is 55–70%.

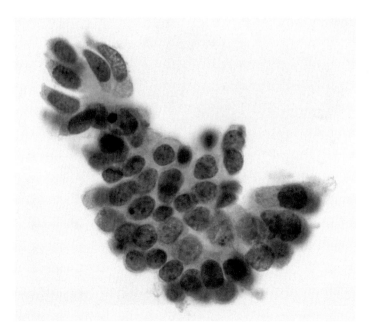

Fig. 14.6. Atypical glandular cells, atypical endocervical cells, favor neoplastic. Sheet of endocervical cells with peripheral palisading of nuclei. This was the only abnormality in this Pap. test. Compare with Fig. 14.9 (ThinPrep; Papanicolaou stain).

Similarities Between AIS and SIL (Table 1)

- Etiologically, both AIS and SIL are associated with HPV 18 or 16.
- AIS and SIL share risk factors such as, oral contraceptive use, multiple sexual partners, early age at first intercourse, and low socioeconomic status.
- AIS is associated with SIL in approx 25–50% of cases (Table 1).

Cytomorphology of AIS

- Increased cellularity.
- Disorderly arranged columnar cells in:
  - Hyperchromatic crowded groups.
  - 2D sheets with honeycomb pattern.
  - Rosettes or acini.
  - Strips with pseudostratification.
  - Single cells.
  - Peripheral nuclear palisading (feathering).
- Nuclei, enlarged to two to three times the size of normal endocervical cells (mean 75 µm^2) variable, round-oval, crowded, altered polarity.
- Nuclear membrane irregularities.
- Chromatin is even with coarse granularity.
- Nucleoli are small.
- Cytoplasm is columnar, finely vacuolated, and amphophilic to cyanophilic.

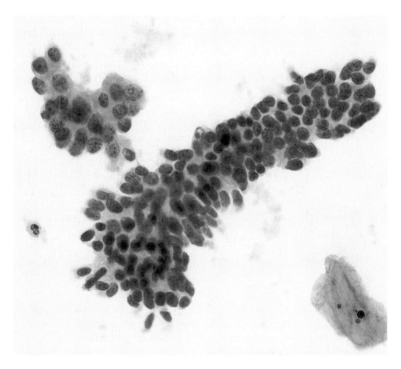

Fig. 14.7. Adenocarcinoma *in situ* with "feathering" (ThinPrep; Papanicolaou stain).

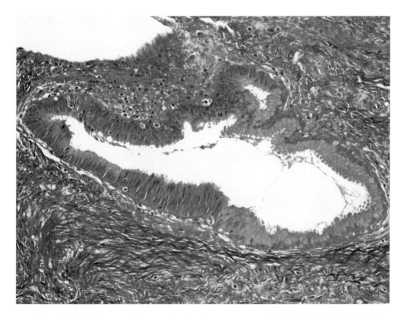

Fig. 14.8. Adenocarcinoma *in situ*. Same case as in Fig. 14.6 (H&E stain).

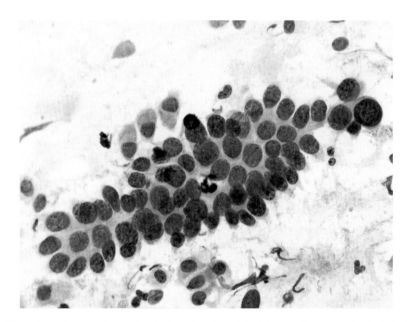

Fig. 14.9. Adenocarcinoma *in situ* in a flat sheet. Nuclei are enlarged with stippled chromatin. Compare to Atypical glandular cells, atypical endocervical cells seen in Fig. 14.6 (conventional smear; Papanicolaou stain).

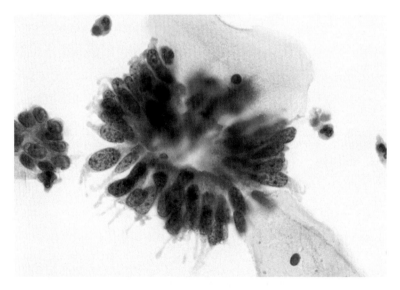

Fig. 14.10. Adenocarcinoma *in situ* with "rosette" and "feathering." Compare the chromatin with that seen in Fig. 14.9 (SurePath; Papanicolaou stain).

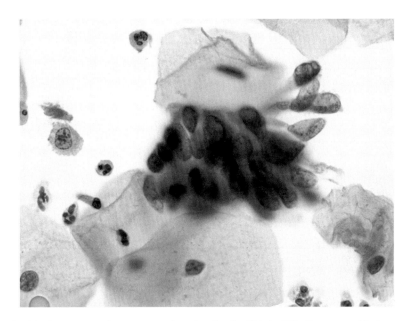

Fig. 14.11. Adenocarcinoma *in situ* in strip of cells ("bird tail"). Compare with the appearance in Fig. 14.12 (SurePath; Papanicolaou stain).

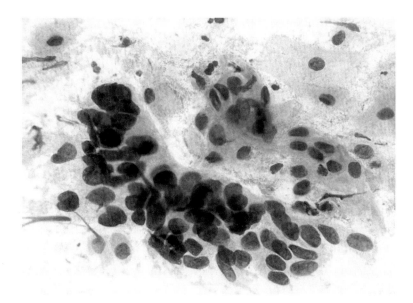

Fig. 14.12. Adenocarcinoma *in situ* in a strip of cells. Compare with the appearance in Fig. 14.11 (conventional smear; Papanicolaou stain).

Table 1
Differences Between AIS and SIL

Features	AIS	SIL
Prevalence	Much less (ranges from 1:26 to 1:237)	Much higher
Mean age	28.8 years	35–39 years
HPV	Predominantly HPV 18	Predominantly HPV 16
Origin	Surface epithelium and superficial glands in TZ	TZ
Colposcopy	Difficult to detect	Easily visualized
Cytologically	Difficult to diagnose	Easier to diagnose
Cytomorphology	Hyperchromatic crowded Groups, strips, rosettes, "feathering," mitoses apoptosis	Single cells, sheets and syncytia mitoses +/–

HPV, human papillomavirus; TZ, transition zone.

- High n:c.
- Mitosis and apoptosis.
- Background inflammatory.
- SIL in approx 50%.
- LBP may show more cellular overlap and smaller strips (bird tail-like).

Differential Diagnosis of AIS on Pap Test (Figs. 14.13–14.18; Tables 2–5)

- HSIL/squamous-cell carcinoma *in situ*.
- Oversampling of endocervix.
- Tubal metaplasia.
- Endometrial cells from lower uterine segment.
- Reactive changes from prior procedure, e.g., cone biopsy.
- Microglandular hyperplasia.
- Rectovaginal fistula.
- Vaginal adenosis.
- Exodus.

HIGH-GRADE SQUAMOUS INTRA-EPITHELIAL LESION

- Involvement of the endocervical gland with HSIL may mimic a glandular lesion.
- Approximately 40% of glandular atypia is HSIL on subsequent biopsy.
- Commonly seen with broom and endocervical brush devices.
- It is seen as hyperchromatic crowded groups, with irregular hyperchromatic nuclei that appear spindled and flattened toward the periphery.
- Nucleoli may be seen.
- Cytoplasm is granular.
- HSIL is distinguished from AIS by the presence of syncytia and single dysplastic cells and lack of "feathering."

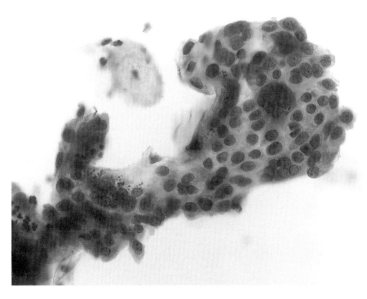

Fig. 14.13. Reactive endocervical cells with enlarged atypical nuclei may mimic endocervical neoplasia. Note that a few atypical nuclei are seen in a sheet of benign-appearing endocervical cells (ThinPrep; Papanicolaou stain).

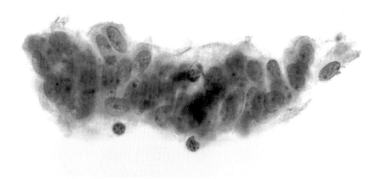

Fig. 14.14. Tubal metaplasia of endocervical cells may show nuclear atypia. Presence of cilia or terminal bar may prevent a false-positive diagnosis (ThinPrep; Papanicolaou stain).

OVERSAMPLING OF ENDOCERVIX

- Can occur from aggressive use of the endocervical brush.
- Shows 2D sheets or clusters of normal columnar ECs with peripheral cellular palisading that mimics "feathering."
- However, in benign ECs the protruding cells show a rim of cytoplasm.

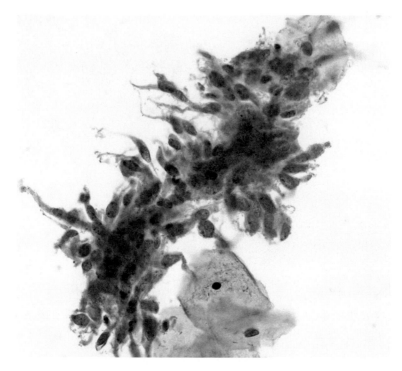

Fig. 14.15. Stromal cells in endocervical polyp are elongated and mimic "feathering." The nuclei, however, are bland and not peripherally oriented (ThinPrep; Papanicolaou stain).

TUBAL METAPLASIA

- Single cells, small groups, pseudostratified strips, or hyperchromatic-crowded groups.
- Cilia or terminal bar present.
- Nuclei are round to oval, enlarged, mildly hyperchromatic, usually centrally located, and nucleoli are not seen.
- Cytoplasm is glandular with discrete vacuoles, or with goblet cell change (peg cells).
- High n:c.
- Mitoses are rare.
- Apoptosis may be seen.

LOWER UTERINE SEGMENT (FIG. 14.19)

- May result from aggressive endocervical sampling or cervical endometriosis.
- Large, thick, tightly packed, more 2D groups of normal endometrial cells with an orderly arrangement of cells.
- Stromal cells are on the outside of the cluster.
- Resulting from cellular crowding, individual cells are difficult to visualize and 3D clusters are not seen as these are not spontaneously exfoliated endometrial cells.

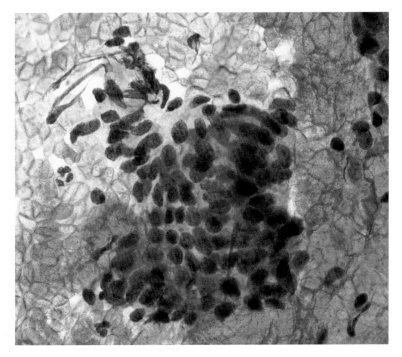

Fig. 14.16. Postcone changes in endocervical cells may mimic endocervical neoplasia because of mild cellular crowding and "feathering." The nuclei, however, are small and lack atypia (conventional smear; Papanicolaou stain).

REACTIVE ECs

- May be seen after conization or radiation.
- Shows slightly to moderately enlarged nuclei with prominent nucleoli and multinucleation.

POSTCONE ECs

- Crowded glandular cells.
- High n:c.
- Nuclei are small, hyperchromatic, and uniform with fine chromatin.
- Endometrial stromal-type cells may be seen in the background.
- History of cone biopsy is helpful.

MICROGLANDULAR HYPERPLASIA

- Associated with oral contraceptive use.
- 3D clusters of ECs with microlumina and fenestrations.
- Nuclei show a spectrum of changes ranging from normal to enlarged and atypical.
- Chromatin is fine to dark.

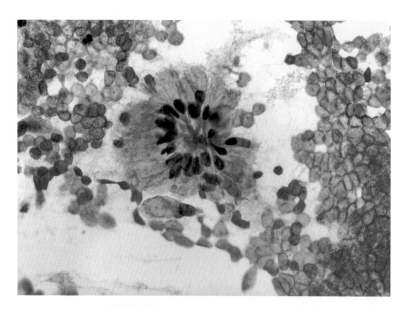

Fig. 14.17. Vaginal adenosis shows mucin-secreting endocervical cells in glandular arrangement (conventional smear; Papanicolaou stain).

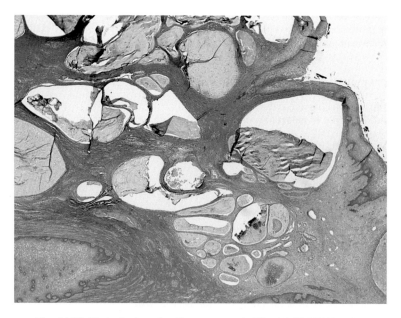

Fig. 14.18. Vaginal adenosis. Same case as in Fig. 14.17 (H&E stain).

Table 2
Reactive Endocervical Cells vs Neoplastic Endocervical Cells

Feature	Reactive	Neoplastic
Architecture	Flat, two dimensional Minimal crowding	Microacini, isolated cells or sheets Crowding, rosettes, strips, "feathering"
Nuclei	Rounded contour	Oval, variable
Anisonucleosis	−	+
Anisocytosis	Rare	Variable, + in higher grade tumors
Nuclear membrane	Smooth	Irregular
Chromatin	Fine	Coarse, hyperchromatic
Nucleoli	+/−, isolated	Usually +, prominent, multiple
Cytoplasm	Cyanophilic, syncytial	Amphophilic or cyanophilic, poorly defined
Background	Clean	Tumor diathesis if invasive carcinoma
Cilia	+	−
Mitosis	−	+
Apoptosis	−	+

Table 3
Tubal Metaplasia vs AIS

Features	Tubal metaplasia	AIS
Architecture	Sheets, strips	Sheets, strips, rosettes, Peripheral nuclear palisading "feathering"
Polarity	Maintained	Disordered arrangement
Nuclei	−	−
Size	Normal to enlarged	Enlarged two-to-three times; normal endocervical cell nuclei
Shape	Round to oval, smooth contour	Elongated and oval, irregular contour
Chromatin	Normal to hyperchromatic, Finely granular	Hyperchromatic, coarsely even; granular, stippled
Nucleoli	Not obvious	+/−

Table 4
Distinguishing Features of HSIL vs AIS

Cells	Syncytial	HSIL
Nuclei	Hyperchromatic	Both
Nucleoli	Micronucleoli	Both
N:c	Increased	Both
"Feathering"	Present	AIS
Apoptosis	Mitoses	AIS

AIS, adenocarcinoma *in situ;* HSIL, high-grade squamous intra-epithelial lesion; n:c, nuclear-to-cytoplasmic ratio.

Table 5
LUS vs AIS

Feature	LUS	AIS
Architecture	Branching tubular glands surrounded by stroma.	Strips, rosettes "feathering"
Cell arrangement	Orderly, overcrowded	Disordered with overlap
Cells	Small (= intermediate cell nucleus)	Columnar or oval
Nuclei	–	–
Size	Small	Enlarged (two to three times intermediate. cell nucleus)
Shape	Round and regular	Columnar to oval, irregular
Chromatin	Compact, uniform, finely granular normal to hyperchromatic	Coarsely granular (stippled) Hyperchromatic
Nucleoli	Usually absent	May be present
Cytoplasm	Scant, eccentric	Scant
Cilia	May be seen	Absent
N:c	Low or high	High
Stroma	Loosely cohesive sheets spindled cells with oval, elongate nuclei	Absent
Mitoses	Present	Present

LUS, lower uterine segment.

- Nucleoli are prominent.
- Cytoplasm shows prominent vacuoles and may mimic adenocarcinoma; however, negative immunostaining with carcinoembryonic antigen is confirmatory of the benign nature of this entity.

RECTOVAGINAL FISTULA

- Cohesive groups and sheets of normal appearing columnar cells with goblet cell differentiation.
- History of rectovaginal fistula may prevent an erroneous diagnosis of atypical or neoplastic glandular cells.

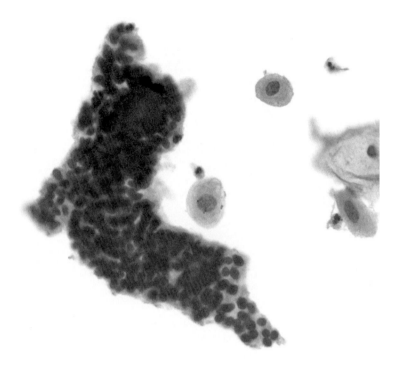

Fig. 14.19. Lower uterine segment. Cohesive group with smooth contour shows small cells with dark uniform nuclei (ThinPrep; Papanicolaou stain).

VAGINAL ADENOSIS

- Replacement of portions of the vaginal squamous mucosa by glandular epithelium.
- May be a precursor to adenocarcinoma of clear-cell type.
- Occurs mainly in women whose mothers received diethylstilbestrol during the first trimester of pregnancy.
- Grossly it appears as a reddish area in the vaginal epithelium.
- Smears show numerous columnar endocervical-type cells dispersed singly, in loosely cohesive groups, or glandular structures.
- Nuclei are located toward the tapered end of the cytoplasm and appear benign.
- Cytoplasm is basophilic and finely vacuolated.

EXODUS

- Menstrual endometrium "exodus" comprises of clustered cells, glandular cells at the edge, and stromal cells at center.
- Glandular cells are cuboidal or cylindrical with vacuolated cytoplasm and small nuclei and nucleoli.
- Stromal cells are tightly packed with barely discernable cytoplasm; stromal cells are CD10 positive and epithelial cells are AE1/AE3-positive.
- Histiocytes are seen, some are hemosiderin-laden.
- Exodus is seen during day 6–10 of the menstrual cycle.

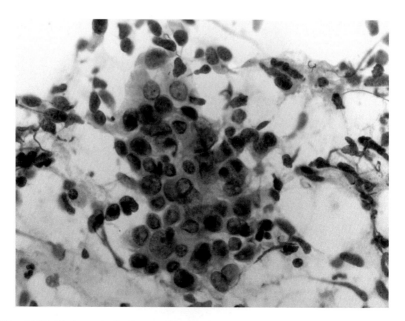

Fig. 14.20. Endocervical adenocarcinoma shows a loosely cohesive group of glandular cells with nuclear atypia, prominent nucleoli, single abnormal cells, and hemorrhagic and necrotic tumor diathesis (conventional smear; Papanicolaou stain).

> ○ *Note: ECs* are rarely seen in "vaginal" smears. After day 12 of the menstrual cycle, *endometrial cells* in a Pap test must be considered abnormal.

ENDOCERVICAL ADENOCARCINOMA (FIGS. 14.20–14.22)

- Comprises up to 25–30% of all cervical carcinoma.
- Frequency is increasing, both relative and absolute.
- High frequency of cervical adenocarcinoma with oral contraceptive use.
- Associated with HPV, mostly HPV 18 particularly, in mucinous and adenosquamous carcinomas.
- Asymptomatic in majority.

Cytomorphology of Endocervical Adenocarcinoma

- High cellularity with dyscohesion and single cells.
- 2D sheets and loosely cohesive clusters.
- Clusters with well-defined scalloped borders.
- Columnar-to-cuboidal cells.
- Loss of polarity.
- Nuclei are enlarged (range: 75 to 150 µm²), crowded, round to oval with pleomorphism, and multinucleation.
- Coarse chromatin, parachromatin clearing.
- Macronucleoli.

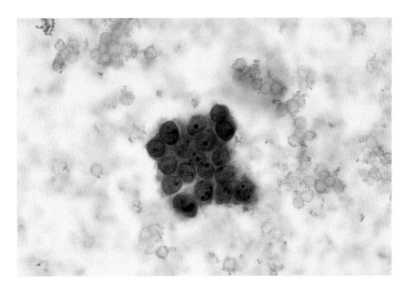

Fig. 14.21. Endocervical adenocarcinoma. Note the well-preserved nuclear features and hemorrhagic tumor diathesis (ThinPrep; Papanicolaou stain).

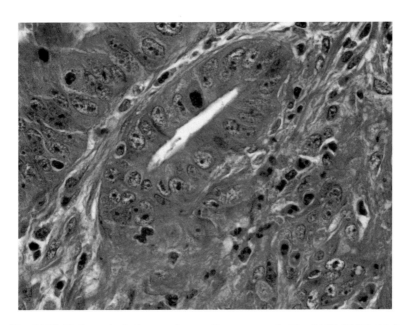

Fig. 14.22. Endocervical adenocarcinoma. Same case as in Fig. 14.21 (H&E stain).

- Cytoplasm has indistinct cell borders, and is foamy or vacuolated.
- Mitoses.
- Hemorrhagic and necrotic tumor diathesis.
- On LBP groups are 3D, nuclear features are crisp with open chromatin, parachromatin clearing and prominent nucleoli.
- More single cells and nuclear contour irregularity.
- On LBP diathesis appears clumped compared with conventional smears where it is diffuse.

Nuclear Features of Endocervical Adenocarcinoma

- Well-defined nuclear membrane   +++*
- Oval nucleus   ++
- Round nucleus   +
- Round nucleolus   +++
- Irregular nuclear shape   +/–
- Multinucleation   +/–

Differential Diagnosis of Adenocarcinoma of the Cervix

- Reactive endocervical cells.
- Repair.
- Lower uterine segment.
- Microglangular hyperplasia.
- Tubal metaplasia.
- Tunnel clusters.
- AIS.
- Metastatic carcinoma.
- Direct extension of endometrial carcinoma.

Variants of Endocervical Adenocarcinoma

- Minimal deviation adenocarcinoma (adenoma malignum).
- Mucinous.
  - Endocervical.
  - Intestinal.
  - Signet ring.
- Endometrioid.
- Clear cell.
- Serous.
- Mesonephric.
- Villoglandular papillary serous.
- Adenosquamous.
- Adenoid cystic.
- Adenoid basal.
- Small-cell variants.

Endocervical Carcinoma vs Endometrial Carcinoma

- Cells from endocervical carcinoma shed more cells than endometrial carcinoma.
- Cells are columnar in endocervical carcinoma and round to oval in endometrial carcinoma.

---

*+++, always present; ++, usually present; +, occasionally present; +/–, may or may not be present.

- Endometrial carcinoma cells are usually arranged in 3D clusters.
- Endocervical carcinoma cells are usually arranged in 2D sheets.
- Cells from endocervical carcinoma are larger.
- Nuclei of endocervical carcinoma cells are larger.
- Cells from endocervical carcinoma more commonly have multiple prominent nucleoli.
- Cytoplasm is more abundant in endocervical carcinoma.
- Cytoplasm in endocervical carcinoma are more amphophilic, whereas cells from endometrial carcinoma are cyanophilic.
- Endometrial cancer usually has a watery background.
- Endocervical cancer has a necrotic hemorrhagic diathesis.
- Apoptosis is more common in endocervical carcinoma.

NOTA BENE

The cytological features of great value in distinguishing benign from neoplastic glandular cells include:

- Nuclear membrane irregularity.
- Multiple and prominent nucleoli.
- Single atypical cells.

15
Endometrial Lesions

INTRODUCTION

- Endometrial carcinoma is the most common malignancy of the gynecological tract.
- An estimated 40,880 new cases of endometrial carcinoma were diagnosed in 2005, and approx 7300 women died of the disease.
- Approximately 80% are adenocarcinomas.
- Incidence of uterine cancer increases after menopause, and approx 75% of cases are diagnosed in postmenopausal patients. The average age at diagnosis is about 60 years.
- Diagnosis of endometrial carcinoma usually depends on clinical signs and symptoms such as abnormal vaginal bleeding; approx 90% are symptomatic.
- The Pap test is not a screening test for endometrial cancer.
- Sensitivity of Pap test for detection of this malignancy is low and varies from 40 to 70% depending on the sampling technique used.
- Pap test sample obtained from posterior cul-de-sac has a detection rate of 60% for endometrial cancer.
- Other more sensitive techniques include endometrial aspiration cytology or endometrial biopsy.
- Specificity of the Pap test is 99.99%. It generally does not lead to a false-positive diagnosis of endometrial adenocarcinoma.

SPONTANEOUSLY EXFOLIATED BENIGN ENDOMETRIAL CELLS IN THE PAP TEST (FIGS. 15.1–15.4)

Epithelial Cells

- Loose clusters and three-dimensional clusters.
- Cells are small, 10–15 μm, cuboidal, or round.
- Nuclei are spherical or oval, 7–10 μm in diameter.
- Occasional tiny nucleoli.
- Chromatin is finely granular.
- Cytoplasm scant and finely vacuolated.

Superficial Stromal Cells (Fig. 15.3)

- Loose aggregates, streaks.
- Resemble histiocytes; cytoplasm is bubbly.
- Nucleus is reniform, round, or oval.

From: *Fundamentals of Pap Test Cytology*
By: R. S. Hoda and S. A. Hoda © Humana Press Inc., Totowa, NJ

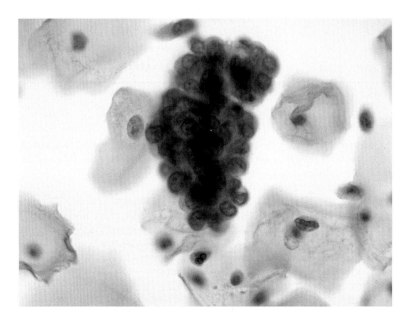

Fig. 15.1. Benign endometrial cells. Three-dimensional clusters of small cells with round nuclei and vacuolated cytoplasm. Occasional nucleoli are seen. Compare with Fig. 15.3 (ThinPrep; Papanicolaou stain).

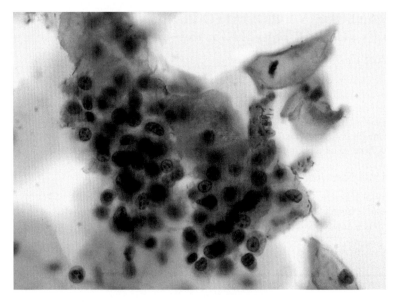

Fig. 15.2. Benign endometrial superficial stromal cells. Loosely cohesive group of round cells with pale, round nuclei and abundant delicate cytoplasm (ThinPrep; Papanicolaou stain).

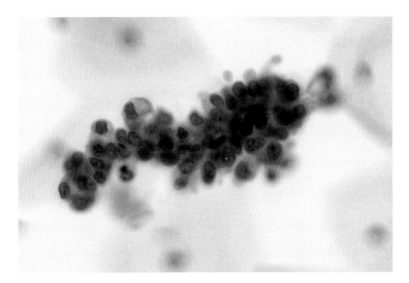

Fig. 15.3. Benign endometrial cells. Cells are similar in morphology to those seen in Fig. 15.1 (SurePath; Papanicolaou stain).

Deep Stromal Cells (Fig. 15.4)

- Loose aggregates of oval-to-spindle shaped.
- Nucleus is small and oval with coarse chromatin.
- Cytoplasm is indistinct.

Differentiating Features of the Two Types of Endometrial Stromal Cells

- Superficial type resemble histiocytes and form loose aggregates.
- Deep stromal cells are round-to-spindle shaped with a small, oval nucleus and scant cytoplasm.

EXODUS (FIGS. 15.5 AND 15.6)

- Occurs on days 6–10 of menstrual cycle.
- Circular cluster of small endometrial stromal cells surrounded by large endometrial epithelial cells.
- Central core formed by the stromal cells is dense and difficult to visualize.
- Stromal cells in the exodus stain positive for CD10, and epithelial cells stain with cytokeratin.

LOWER UTERINE SEGMENT

- Tight groups of two-dimensional fragments of branching tubular glands.
- Stromal cells are on the outside.
- Stromal cells are round to spindled with oval nuclei.
- Capillaries are seen traversing the stroma.
- Glandular cells are small with crowded overlapping reniform nuclei and scant, wispy cytoplasm.

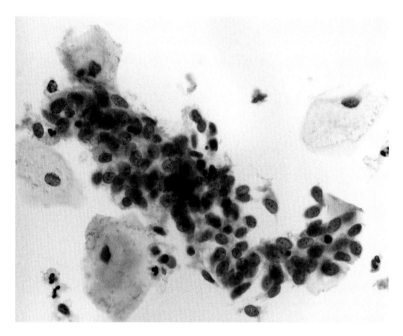

Fig. 15.4. Benign endometrial deep stromal cells. Spindle-shaped cells in a loosely cohesive arrangement. Nuclei are uniform and spindled (ThinPrep; Papanicolaou stain).

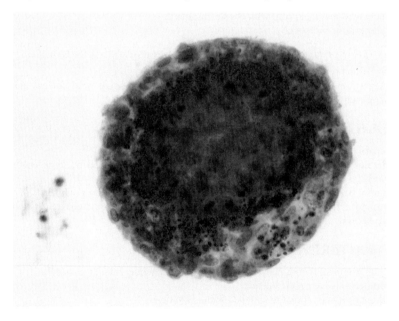

Fig. 15.5. Exodus. Dense core of endometrial epithelial cells surrounded by endometrial stromal cells seen on day 6 of the menstrual cycle. Compare with Fig. 15.6 (ThinPrep; Papanicolaou stain).

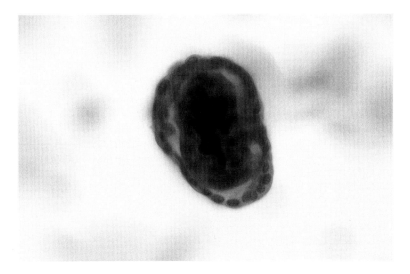

Fig. 15.6. Exodus appears similar to Fig. 15.5 (SurePath; Papanicolaou stain).

- Mitoses.
- Apoptosis.

Differential Diagnosis of Lower Uterine Segment

- Endometriosis.
- Endocervical cells.
- Atrophy.
- Tubal metaplasia.
- Adenocarcinoma *in situ*.
- High-grade squamous intra-epithelial lesion.
- Endometrial carcinoma.

ENDOMETRIAL METAPLASTIC PROCESSES

- Squamous metaplasia is seen in association with endometrial hyperplasia and endometroid carcinoma.
- Papillary syncytial metaplasia show papillary aggregates with fibrovascular cores comprised of eosinophilic cells.
- Tubal metaplasia.
- Eosinophilic metaplasia.

CONDITIONS IN WHICH ENDOMETRIAL CELLS ARE SEEN IN A PAP TEST

- Dysfunctional bleeding.
- Hormonal therapy.
- Intrauterine device (IUD).
- Endometriosis.
- Chronic endometritis.

- Acute and chronic endocervitis.
- Pregnancy.
- Immediate postpartum state.
- Recent endometrial instrumentation.
- Menstrual period.
- Endometrial polyp.
- Submucosal leiomyoma.
- Endometrial hyperplasia, simple, complex, and atypical.
- Endometrial carcinoma.
  - *Note:* In Pap test, the presence of endometrial cells after the 12th day of the menstrual cycle and particularly after menopause are considered abnormal even in the absence of cytological atypia.
- Presence of endometrial cells is related to:
  - Days of menstrual cycle.
  - Collection method and area sampled; spontaneously exfoliated endometrial cells differ from those obtained by scraping or endometrial aspiration.
- Significance of endometrial cells depends on:
  - Age of patient.
  - Last menstrual period.
  - Hormone therapy status.
  - Abnormal uterine bleeding.
  - IUD use.
  - Recent instrumentation.
  - Presence of endometriosis.

Endometrial Cells vs Endocervical Cells

- Endometrial cells are packed together with scant cytoplasm.
- Endocervical cells form looser clusters and are more abundant cytoplasm.

CYTOLOGY OF ATYPICAL ENDOMETRIAL EPITHELIAL CELLS (FIGS. 15.7 AND 15.8)

- Associated with higher rates of carcinoma.
- Small groups are less than 10 cells.
- Slightly enlarged hyperchromatic nucleus.
- Small nucleoli.
- Nuclear atypia is greater than benign reactive or regenerative cells.
- Vacuolated cytoplasm.

Where Atypical Endometrial Cells May be Seen

- Atypical endometrial hyperplasia.
- Endometrial polyp.
- Endometritis.
- Arias–Stella.
- Menstrual smear.
- Hormone therapy in postmenopausal women.

CYTOLOGY OF ENDOMETRIAL HYPERPLASIA

- It shows increased numbers of tight tubular or pseudopapillary clusters of benign endometrial cells.

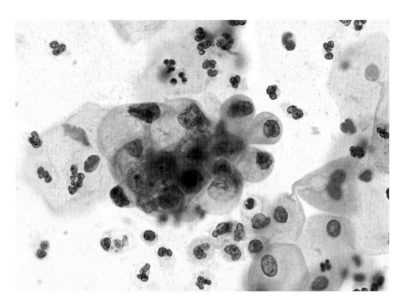

Fig. 15.7. Atypical glandular cells–atypical endometrial cells. Three-dimensional cluster with scalloped borders. Eccentric round-to-reniform nuclei with a moderate amount of vacuolated cytoplasm. Compare with the case of endometrial adenocarcinoma in Figs. 15.10 and 15.12 (conventional smear; Papanicolaou stain).

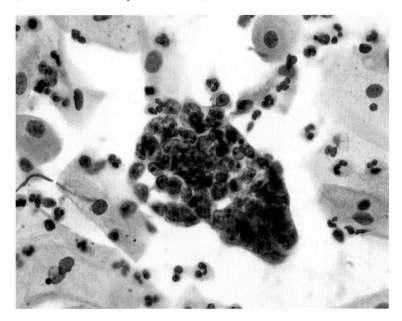

Fig. 15.8. Atypical glandular cells–atypical endometrial cells. The cluster shows cellular overlap and hyperchromatic nuclei. Nuclei are atypical but small. Compare with intermediate cell nuclei (conventional smear; Papanicolaou stain).

- Nuclei are overlapping, slightly enlarged, regular and vesicular, and nucleoli are small.
- Cytoplasm is scant.
  - *Note:* Pap test is not reliable for the diagnosis of endometrial hyperplasia. Diagnosis is reliably rendered on endometrial biopsy or curettage.

Cytology of Atypical Endometrial Hyperplasia

- Cytological changes depend on the severity of atypia.
- Nuclei are enlarged, irregular, and hyperchromatic.
- Nucleoli are present.

VARIANTS OF ENDOMETRIAL ADENOCARCINOMA

- Endometrioid (most common).
  - Secretory.
  - Ciliated.
  - With squamous differentiation.
- Serous.
- Clear cell.
- Mucinous.
- Squamous.
- Undifferentiated.

CYTOLOGY OF ENDOMETRIAL CARCINOMA (FIGS. 15.9–15.16)

Low-Grade Endometrial Carcinoma

- High estrogen effect.
- Few abnormal clusters of tightly packed, loosely cohesive cells.
- Nuclei are enlarged and nucleoli are prominent.
- Cytoplasm is scant and vacuolated.
- Histiocytes with foamy cytoplasm and cytoplasmic neutrophils.
- Watery tumor diathesis.

High-Grade Endometrial Carcinoma

- Moderate-to-high cellularity.
- Clusters and papillary structures of large endometrial cells.
- Nuclei large, hyperchromatic, irregular with multiple nucleoli.
- Cytoplasm is variable and may be abundant and vacuolated.
- Histiocytes with foamy cytoplasm and cytoplasmic neutrophils.
- Tumor diathesis is granular to necrotic depending on tumor grade.

ENDOMETRIAL CARCINOMA WITH MUCINOUS FEATURES (FIGS. 15.17 AND 15.18)

- Is the only variant discussed further because the bland cytological features may lead to a false-negative diagnosis.
- Well-differentaited tumor.
- Clusters of tumor cells with a signet-ring configuration.
- Cytoplasmic vacuoles with mucinous condensation.
- Bland nuclei.
- In patients without a prior history of mucinous endometrial carcinoma, the cytological features may mimic microglandular hyperplasia, endometrial mucinous proliferations.

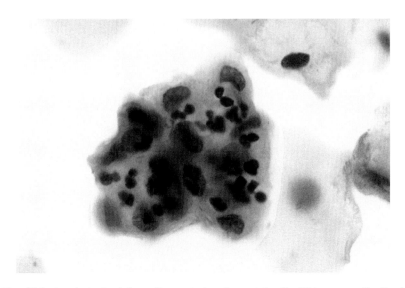

Fig. 15.9. Atypical glandular cells-atypical endometrial cells. This group of cells show intracytoplasmic neutrophils and was the only such group in this Pap from a 65-year-old woman (ThinPrep; Papanicolaou stain).

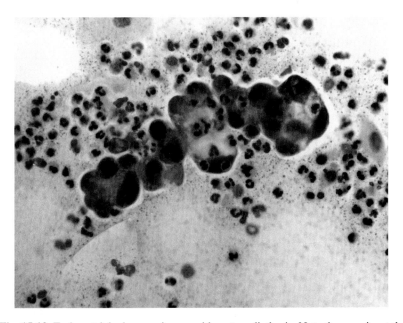

Fig. 15.10. Endometrial adenocarcinoma with watery diathesis. Note the prominent three-dimensional cluster of endometrial cells with enlarged hyperchromatic nuclei. Vacuolated cytoplasm indents some nuclei (conventional smear; Papanicolaou stain).

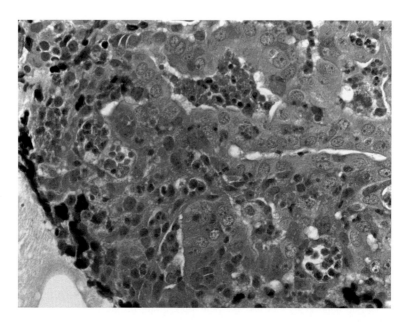

Fig. 15.11. Endometrial adenocarcinoma. Same case as in Fig. 15.10 (H&E stain).

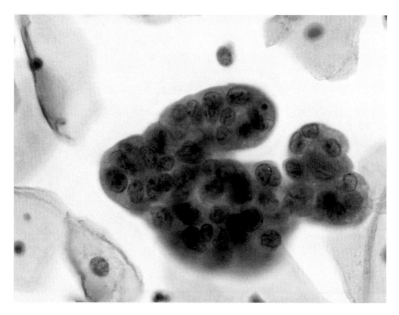

Fig. 15.12. Endometrial adenocarcinoma. Three-dimensional cluster of endometrial cells with slight nuclear enlargement, more open chromatin, and small nucleoli. Compare with Fig. 15.13 (SurePath; Papanicolaou stain).

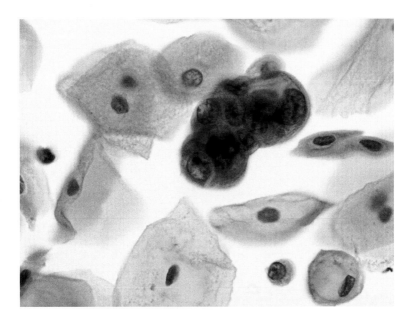

Fig. 15.13. Endometrial adenocarcinoma. Note the nuclear enlargement and irregularity in shape. Compare with Fig. 15.12 (SurePath; Papanicolaou stain).

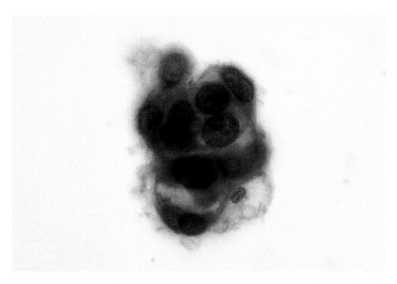

Fig. 15.14. Endometrial adenocarcinoma. Note the distinct cytoplasmic vacuole (ThinPrep; Papanicolaou stain).

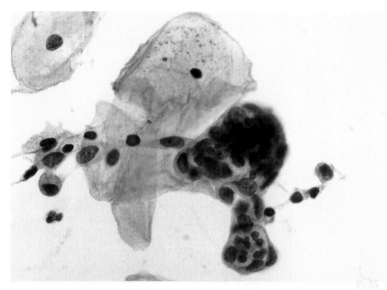

Fig. 15.15. Endometrial adenocarcinoma. Note the distinct cytoplasmic vacuole with intact intracytoplasmic neutrophils (ThinPrep; Papanicolaou stain).

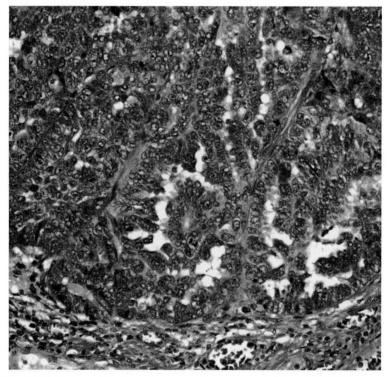

Fig. 15.16. Endometrial adenocarcinoma. Same case as in Fig. 15.17 (H&E stain).

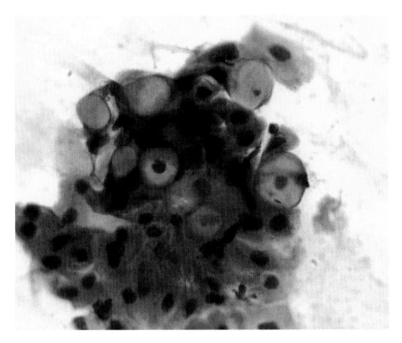

Fig. 15.17. Recurrent endometrial adenocarcinoma, mucinous type. Cluster of cells with signet-ring morphology. Cytoplasm shows mucinous condensation. This may lead to an erroneous diagnosis of treatment-associated changes (conventional smear; Papanicolaou stain).

- Recurrent mucinous endometrial carcinoma may be difficult to distinguish cytologically from radiation effect.

THE DIFFERENTIAL DIAGNOSIS OF ENDOMETRIAL CARCINOMA

Note that a Pap smear should not be viewed as a method to screen for endometrial carcinoma.

Neoplastic

- Endocervical adenocarcinoma (Table 1).
- Other gynecological malignancies (fallopian tubes*, ovary*, vagina).
- Adenocarcinoma from other sites (breast, colon, bladder).
- Nonkeratinizing squamous cell carcinoma.
- Adenocarcinoma *in situ.*

Nonneoplastic

- Endocervical cells with tubal metaplasia.

---

*All these entities, neoplastic and nonneoplastic, may be morphologically indistinguishable from endometrial carcinoma. Clinical history may be helpful.

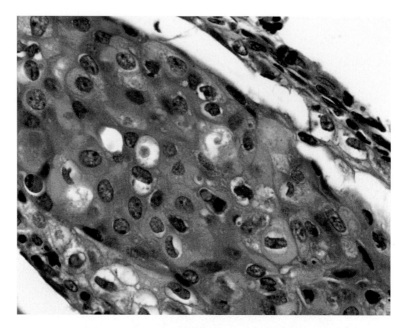

Fig. 15.18. Primary endometrial adenocarcinoma, mucinous type—same case as in Fig. 15.17 (H&E stain).

Table 1
Endocervical Carcinoma vs Endometrial Carcinoma

Feature	Endocervical carcinoma	Endometrial carcinoma
Cellularity	++	+
Diathesis	Necrotic	Watery diathesis
Cell size	Large, ~190 μm²	Smaller, 140 μm²
Cell shape	Columnar	Rounder
Architecture	Sheets, single	Clusters, single
Histiocytes	Not usually seen	Commonly seen
Nuclear size	Large, ~90 μm²	Smaller, 60 μm²
Cytoplasm	Amphophilic	Cyanophilic
N:c ratio	Lower	Higher
Nucleoli	++	+
Cells	Columnar	Round-oval
Cell arrangement	Two-dimensional	Three-dimensional
Papillae	++	−
Strips	+	−
Apoptosis	+	+/−
Associated SIL	++	−

n:c, nuclear-to-cytoplasmic ratio; SIL, squamous intra-epithelial lesion.
−, absent; +, present; ++, common.

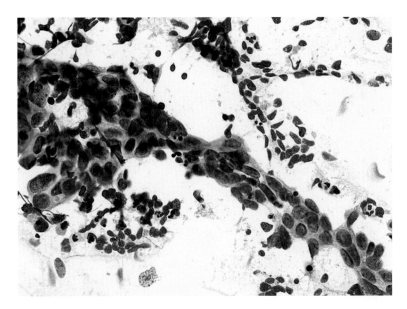

Fig. 15.19. Malignant epithelial component in a malignant mixed Mullerian tumor. Note the necrotic tumor diathesis in the background of malignant epithelial cells (conventional smear; Papanicolaou stain).

- Endometrial cells with papillary syncytial metaplasia.
- Microglandular hyperplasia*.
- Endometrial hyperplasia.
- Endometrial polyp.
- Pemphigus vulgaris.
- IUD*.
- Arias–Stella reaction*.

NONEPITHELIAL UTERINE TUMORS

Nonepithelial tumors can be either primary, direct extensions from the vagina or the uterus, or metastatic to the cervix.

Benign

- Leiomyoma.
- Endometrial stromal tumor.

Malignant (Figs. 15.19 and 15.20)

- Malignant mixed Mullerian tumor.
- Leiomyosarcoma.
- Endometrial stromal tumor.

---

*All these entities, neoplastic and nonneoplastic, may be morphologically indistinguishable from endometrial carcinoma. Clinical history may be helpful in differential diagnosis.

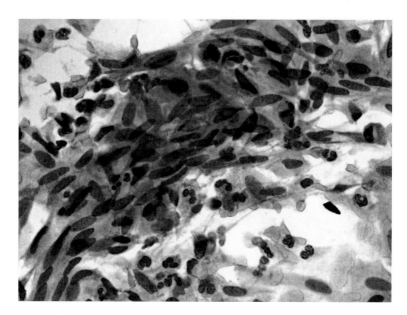

Fig. 15.20. Leiomyosarcoma with fascicles of spindle-shaped cells with long ill-defined cytoplasmic processes. Nuclei are cigar-shaped and hyperchromatic (conventional smear; Papanicolaou stain).

- Malignant lymphoma and leukemia.
- Malignant melanoma.
- Trophoblastic tumors.

ARIAS–STELLA REACTION (FIG. 15.21)

The Arias–Stella reaction is one of the cytological findings in pregnancy characterized by presence of:

- Atypical large endometrial cells with hyperchromatic nuclei.
- Prominent nucleoliabundant, vacuolated cytoplasm.
- Nuclear-to-cytoplamic ratio is low.
- Morphologically difficult to distinguish from endometrial carcinoma.
  - Please *see* Chapter 6.

BENIGN APPEARING ENDOMETRIAL CELLS IN A WOMAN 40 OR OLDER: OTHER CATEGORY

- The 2001 Bethesda system recommends the reporting of all benign-appearing endometrial cells (BAEMC) (glandular cells only) in women 40 years of age or older, irrespective of menstrual or hormone replacement therapy status.
- With Bethesda 2001 the percentage of Pap tests with BAEMC showed a fivefold increase.
- BAEMC on Paps in women 40 or older may indicate endometrial pathology in 35–40% of women including hyperplasia, polyp, submucosal leiomyoma, or adenocarcinoma.

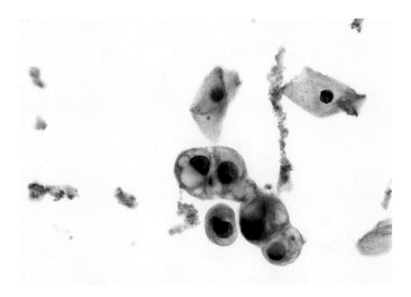

Fig. 15.21. Arias–Stella reaction. Vacuolated cytoplasm with small eccentric nuclei. Compare with Fig. 15.10 (ThinPrep; Papanicolaou stain).

- The risk of endometrial adenocarcinoma with BAEMC on Paps of women 40 years or older depends on age and menopausal status. The rates of cancer have been found to be 2% in 40–50 year olds, 4% in 50–59 year olds, and 13–17% in those older than 59 years.
- The majority of endometrial adenocarcinomas are symptomatic; however, 10–25% are asymptomatic and may come to clinical attention on the bases of cytological finding of BAEMC in Pap test.
- A meta-analysis found that 6% of postmenopausal women with BAEMC have endometrial carcinoma on subsequent biopsy.

Causes of Benign Glandular Cells in Posthysterectomy Women

- Uterine prolapse.
- Vaginal endometriosis.
- Fistula.
- Vaginal adenosis not associated with diethylstilbestrol exposure.
- Glandular metaplasia associated with prior radiation or chemotherapy.
  - *Note:* Endometrial carcinoma cells are best detected in a sample from the vaginal fornix.

MIMICS OF ENDOMETRIAL CELLS

- Follicular cervicitis.
- "Bare" nuclei seen in atrophy.
- Small, blue cells seen with tamoxifen treatment (Fig. 15.22).
- Atrophic endocervical cells.
- Squamous pearls with swirling of cells.

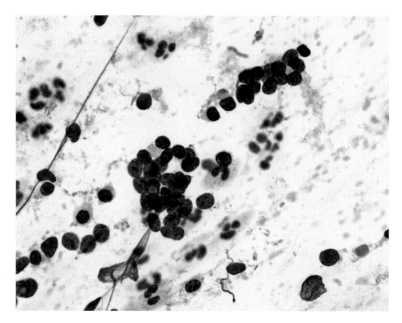

Fig. 15.22. Reserve cells in tamoxifen treatment (tamoxifen cells). Small, dark, and uniform "bare" nuclei. Distinguished from endometrial carcinoma by the lack of cytoplasm and uniformity of nuclei, and from small-cell carcinoma by lack of cytoplasm and background necrosis (conventional smear; Papanicolaou stain).

HISTIOCYTES IN PAP TEST (FIG. 15.23)

- There is no significant association between the presence of histiocytes alone and endometrial carcinoma. Histiocytes alone, in the absence of postmenopausal bleeding and endometrial cells (benign appearing or atypical), are a poor indicator of endometrial pathology.
- Presence of both endometrial cells and histiocytes particularly, in a postmenopausal woman, have a sensitivity and specificity of 82 and 67% for detecting endometrial carcinoma.
- Clinical suspicion of endometrial cancer and atypia of endometrial cells are more predictive of endometrial carcinoma.
- Cytologically, the histiocytes are large and vacuolated with engulfed intracytoplasmic neutrophils.

NOTA BENE

- In Pap tests, increased squamous cell maturation (high levels of estrogenic activity) after menopause may be associated with endometrial pathology.
- Benign-appearing endometrial cells on Pap smears of premenopausal women younger than 40 years of age are rarely associated with endometrial adenocarcinoma.
- Metastatic lobular carcinomas of breast are in the differential diagnosis of endometrial carcinoma (Fig. 15.24).

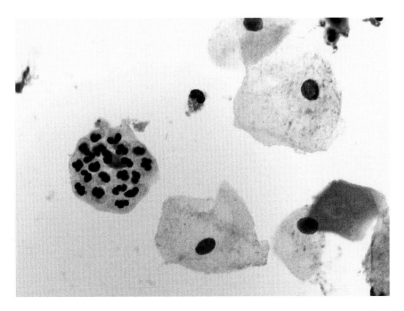

Fig. 15.23. Histiocytes. Small pale nucleus and numerous ingested neutrophils (ThinPrep; Papanicolaou stain).

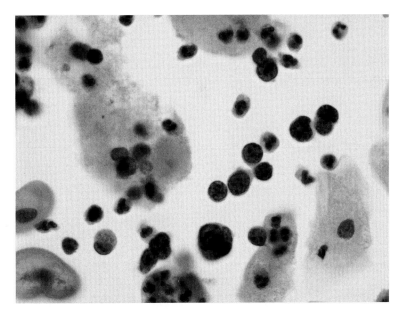

Fig. 15.24. Metastatic lobular carcinoma of the breast in a Pap smear. Note the linear cell arrangement. Distinguished from endometrial carcinoma by the small cell size, high nuclear-to-cytoplasmic ratio, and arrangement of cells (ThinPrep; Papanicolaou stain).

16
Metastatic Tumors

NOTABLE POINTS REGARDING DETECTION OF METASTATIC TUMORS IN THE PAP TEST

- Samples: Obtained from the vaginal fornix rather than the cervix and have a better yield in detecting metastatic malignant cells, as these cells are shed in the vaginal fornix.
- Incidence: 11 extrauterine malignancies are seen for every 100,000 (0.4%) Pap tests screened. One extrauterine malignancy is detected on the Pap test for every seven uterine cancers detected. Approximately 50% of metastatic tumors seen in a Pap test are of gynecological origin, and approx 50% are of nongynecological origin.
- Features influencing detection of metastatic tumor in the Pap test: Include the type of sampling method used, extent and location of the tumor, and tumor grade.

Pap tests with metastatic tumors typically have a cleaner background, and usually the necrotic and hemorrhagic diathesis of primary cervical tumors or the watery diathesis of endometrial carcinomas is absent. Metastatic colon carcinomas or high-grade endometrial and ovarian carcinomas may show necrotic diathesis.

In some cases, the presence of metastatic tumor cells may be the first sign of malignancy and should be promptly followed up. Presence of metastatic tumor in the Pap test may be used for tumor staging and clinical management. Misdiagnosis of a metastatic carcinoma as a primary uterine tumor may lead to unnecessary surgery.

The most common metastatic tumors to the female genital tract include breast carcinoma and carcinomas of the endometrium (Figs. 16.1–16.3), ovary, colon, and urinary bladder (please *see* Chapter 15 for endometrial carcinoma).

CYTOMORPHOLOGY OF SEROUS OVARIAN CARCINOMA (FIGS. 16.4 AND 16.5)

- Three-dimensional clusters.
- Large cells.
- Nuclei are large with macronucleoli.
- Cytoplasm is variable in amount and may be vacuolated.
- Psammoma bodies may be present.
- May simulate high-grade endometrial or fallopian tube carcinomas.

Psammoma Bodies (Fig. 16.4)

- Are small spherical structures calcified in concentric layers.
- Usually stain blue.

From: *Fundamentals of Pap Test Cytology*
By: R. S. Hoda and S. A. Hoda © Humana Press Inc., Totowa, NJ

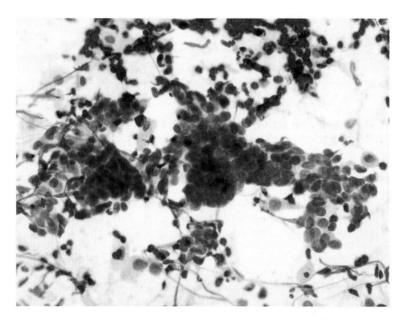

Fig. 16.1. Metastatic serous adenocarcinoma of the endometrium in a Pap smear. Hyperchromatic crowded group of endometrial cells and single malignant cells. Compare with Fig. 16.3 (conventional smear; Papanicolaou stain).

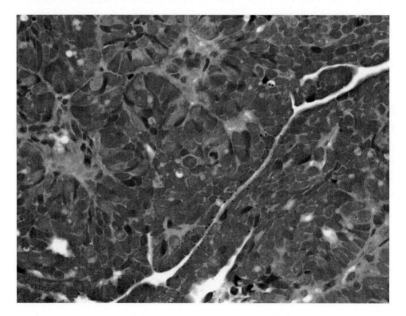

Fig. 16.2. Primary serous adenocarcinoma of the endometrium. The same case as shown in Fig. 16.1 (H&E stain).

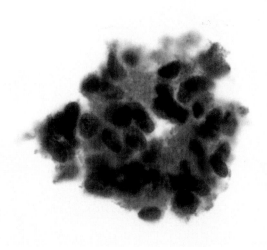

Fig. 16.3. Metastatic adenocarcinoma of the endometrium in a Pap smear. Note the clean background. Compare with Fig. 16.1 (ThinPrep; Papanicolaou stain).

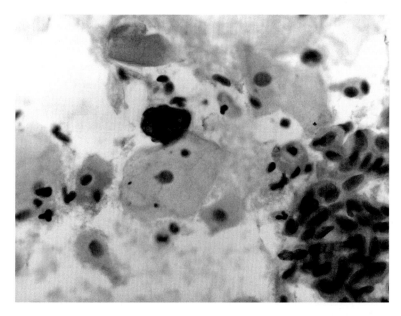

Fig. 16.4. Psammoma body as the only "finding" in a case of ovarian serous carcinoma (conventional smear; Papanicolaou stain).

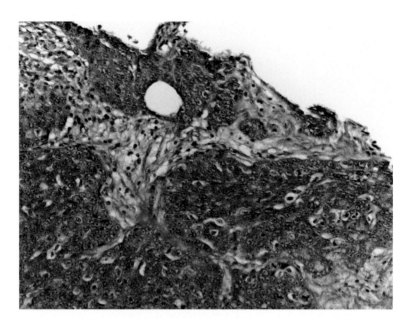

Fig. 16.5. Primary ovarian serous carcinoma. The same case as shown in Fig 16.4 also showed rare psammoma bodies (H&E stain).

- May appear isolated or found in the center of cancer cells.
- Psammoma bodies accompanied by large tumor cells usually suggest a serous tumor of the ovary, and rarely endometrium or fallopian tube origin and neuroendocrine carcinoma of the cervix.
- It may also be associated with nonneoplastic conditions such as endosalpingiosis.
- Calcified debris in women with intrauterine device may mimic psammoma bodies.

METASTATIC DUCTAL CARCINOMA OF THE BREAST (FIG. 16.6)

- Extremely rare with a only a few reported cases.
- Cytological features depend on histological grade and type of mammary primary.
- Metastases in a Pap smear are usually indicative of widespread disease and poor prognosis.

METASTATIC MERKEL-CELL CARCINOMA (FIGS. 16.7 AND 16.8)

- Extremely rare with only one reported case of cervicovaginal metastatsis in a patient with widespread disease.
- Small-to-medium-sized cells in a predominantly discohesive or single-cell pattern. The nuclei were uniform, round to oval, with delicate nuclear membranes. The chromatin pattern was fine. The cytoplasm was very scanty. Intermediate filament "buttons" were abundant. Rare rosette formation. Mitoses and apoptosis are present. Differential diagnosis includes other small cell tumors. Immunocytochemistry and review of the primary tumor may be useful.

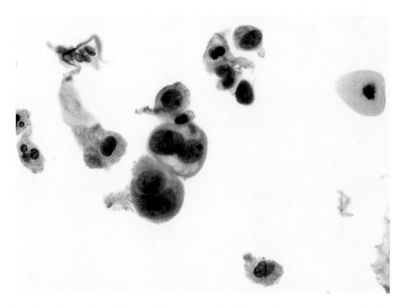

Fig. 16.6. Metastatic carcinoma of the breast, ductal type in Pap smear. Note the large cells with round nuclei and promiment nucleoli. Cytoplasm is delicate. Cell-in-cell configuration is also seen. Compare with Figs. 16.1 and 16.3 (ThinPrep; Papanicolaou stain).

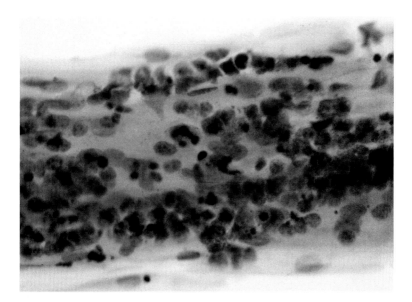

Fig. 16.7. Metastatic Merkel carcinoma in a Pap smear. Numerous single cells with vague nuclear molding and washed-out chromatin. Paranuclear "buttons" are seen. Cytoplasm is ill-defined (conventional smear; Papanicolaou stain).

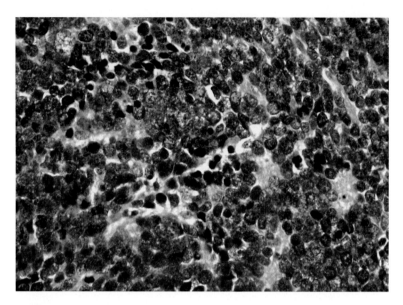

Fig. 16.8. Primary Merkel carcinoma of the skin of the thigh. The same case as shown in Fig. 16.7 (H&E stain).

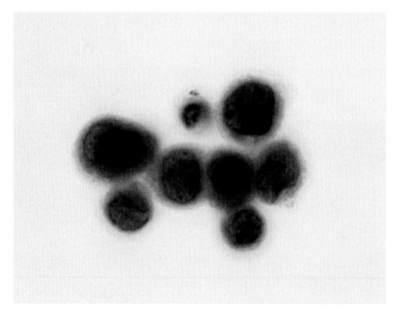

Fig. 16.9. Metastatic carcinoma of the breast, lobular type in a Pap smear. Note the round cells with eccentric irregular nuclei and small nucleoli (ThinPrep; Papanicolaou stain).

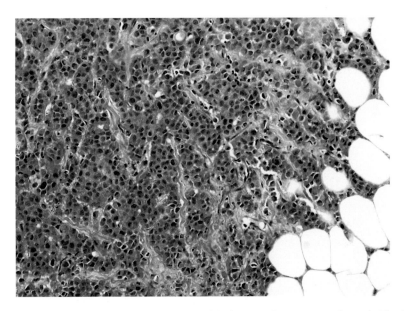

Fig. 16.10. Primary carcinoma of the breast, lobular type. Same case as shown in Fig. 16.9 (H&E stain).

METASTATIC LOBULAR CARCINOMA OF THE BREAST (FIGS. 16.9 AND 16.10)

- Cells are small, with some in signet-ring forms*.
- Arranged as single cells in linear files ("Indian filing") and loosely cohesive groups.
- Nuclei are small, dark, irregular and peripherally located.
- Cytoplasm is vacuolated with mucinous condensation ("targetoid body").
- Metastatic lobular carcinoma may mimic high-grade squamous intra-epithelial lesion or endometrial carcinoma.

---

*Signet-ring cells are characteristic of mammanl lobular carcinoma, although cytologically similar cells may be seen in metastatic gastric carcinoma.

17
Therapy-Related Changes

COMMON AGENTS THAT CAUSE IATROGENIC CHANGES IN PAP SMEARS

- Chemotherapy.
- Cautery.
- Intrauterine device, diaphragm, pessary.
- Laser.
- Postinstrumentation: biopsy.
- Radiation therapy.

CYTOLOGICAL FEATURES OF RADIATION THERAPY (FIG. 17.1)

- Cytomegaly.
- Karyomegaly.
- Normal nuclear-to-cytoplasmic (n:c) ratio.
- Bizarre cell shape.
- Multinucleation.
- Nuclear wrinkling and smudging.
- Altered nuclear and cytoplasmic staining.
- Nuclear and cytoplasmic vacuolization.
- Intracytoplasmic neutrophils.

Acute Radiation Changes (Fig. 17.2)

- Large cell with normal n:c ratio.
- Nuclear membrane is irregular.
- Multinucleation is common.
- Pleomorphism.
- Dirty background.
- Leukophagocytosis.
- Smudged nuclear chromatin.
- Cytoplasmic vacuoles.

Chronic Radiation Change

- Some changes of acute radiation effect persist.
- Pale smudged nuclei.

From: *Fundamentals of Pap Test Cytology*
By: R. S. Hoda and S. A. Hoda © Humana Press Inc., Totowa, NJ

Table 1
Radiation Atypia vs Squamous Intra-Epithelial Lesion

	Radiation	Squamous intra-epithelial lesion
Cells	Single/loose aggregates	Single/aggregates
Size of cells	Large	–
N:c	Normal	Increased
Nucleus	Dark, vacuolated	Hyperchromatic
	Rnlarged, multiple	Enlarged
Nuclear Contour	Smooth	Irregular
Nucleoli	+	–
Cytoplasm	Vacuolated	Granular

–, absent; +, present.

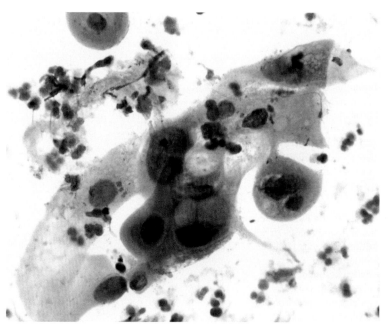

Fig. 17.1. Radiation effect in a Pap smear. "Streaming" sheet of enlarged cells and low nuclear-to-cytoplasmic ratio. Nuclei are enlarged with prominent nucleoli and binucleation, and cytoplasm shows distinct vacuoles. Polychromasia was seen. Compare with Fig. 17.2 (conventional smear; Papanicolaou stain).

- Low n:c ratio.
- Biphasic (psychedelic) cytoplasmic staining.
- Changes of repair and regeneration.
- Liquid-based preparations show less psychedelic staining.

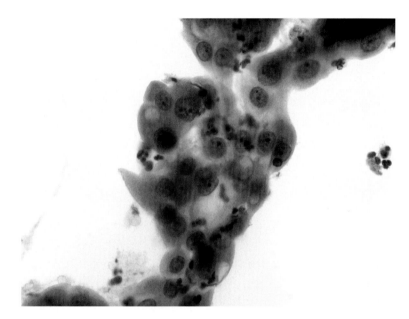

Fig. 17.2. Radiation effect in a Pap smear. The cells, although "streaming," have a more rounded contour. Compare with Fig. 17.1 (ThinPrep; Papanicolaou stain).

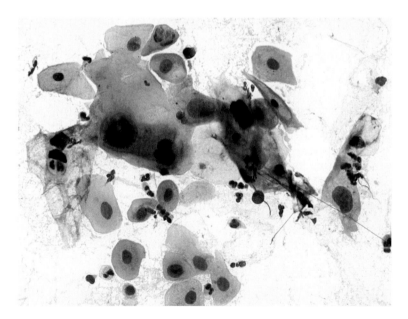

Fig. 17.3. Radiation-associated atypia. Large cells with large hyperchromatic atypical nuclei. Occasional cells show high nuclear-to-cytoplasmic ratio. Compare with Figs. 17.1 and 17.2 (conventional smear; Papanicolaou stain).

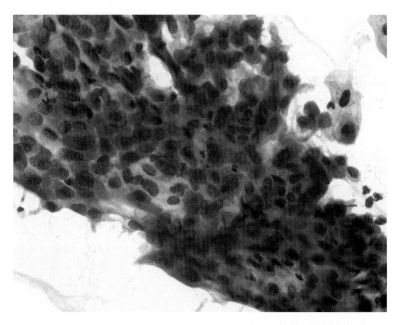

Fig. 17.4. Recurrent squamous-cell carcinoma, status-post radiation. Cohesive sheet of disorganized cells with nuclear overlap and hyperchromatism and high nuclear-to-cytoplasmic ratio. Compare with Figs. 17.1 and 17.2 (ThinPrep; Papanicolaou stain).

POSTRADIATION ATYPIA/DYSPLASTIC CHANGES (FIG. 17.3)

- Atypia or dysplastic changes status-post radiation may be difficult to distinguish from reactive changes (Table 1).
- Prognostic significance of cytologically detected atypia or dysplastic changes is uncertain.
- Sampling of ulcerated areas may show reactive changes in the epithelium and the stroma that may mimic recurrent disease.
- Cells are enlarged, cytoplasmic vacuolation +/–, nuclei are hyperchromatic (some of "India ink" quality) with contour irregularity, multinucleation, and high n:c.

RECURRENT CARCINOMA S/P RADIATION (FIG. 17.4)

- All features of malignancy.
- Review of pathology from primary tumor would be prudent.

GLANDULAR CELLS, S/P HYSTERECTOMY, POSSIBLE ORIGINS

- Fistula.
- Vaginal adenosis.
- Endometriosis.

- Prolapsed fallopian tubes.
- Supracervical hysterectomy.
- Glandular metaplasia following radiation or chemotherapy.

SIGNIFICANCE AND MORPHOLOGY OF "TAMOXIFEN" CELLS

- Present in 40% of Pap smears in women on tamoxifen.
- Non-neoplastic in nature.
- Could represent proliferative reserve cells of cervical–vaginal epithelium.
- Probably result from estrogenic effect of tamoxifen on cervical–vaginal epithelium.
- Small, tightly cohesive clusters of cells.
- Cells have scant-to-absent cytoplasm.
- Nuclei are similar to intermediate squamous cells with a smooth nuclear membrane.
- Fine, hyperchromatic chromatin and indistinct, minute nucleoli.

18

Artifacts, Contaminants, and Incidental Findings

Common Pap Test Artifacts

Air-drying artifact: predominantly seen in conventional smears and result in polychromatic staining, cellular and nuclear enlargement (Fig. 18.1).

Brown artifact: "corn flakes," air-trapping under cover slip—"brown cell" artifact (Fig. 18.2).

Brush artifact: glandular crowding; aggressive sampling via an endocervix brush.

Lubricating jelly: may contaminate Pap smears; amorphous material with a blue tinge.

Contaminants in Pap test: contaminants may be intrinsic or extrinsic.

Extrinsic: are more common and presumably derived from the tap water used in the Papanicolaou staining procedure, in the air or on the hands of the laboratory technician.

Intrinsic: are less common (e.g., air-drying: "corn flakes"; Table 1).

Additional Contaminants in the Pap Test

Alternaria: brown color, segmented body, likened to "snowshoe" (Fig. 18.3).

Aspergillus **spp.:** may be a contaminant in a Pap or may represent an active infection in people on prolonged antibiotic treatment or in immunocompromised women with isolated cutaneous aspergillosis of the labia minora. The fungi form a conidial head or a "fruiting body" that produces spores in cavities (aspergilloma). The fruiting body is important in aspergillus species identification and in distinguishing the fungus from its mimics, such as *Zygomycetes* and *Candida* spp. (Fig. 18.4).

Insects (arthropods): appearance depends on the insect and the body part seen.

Ova of *Enterobius vermicularis* (also known as a pinworm or roundworm): ovum of *E. vermicularis* are the most common ova to be seen in a Pap test. These have elongated oval shapes with flattening of the ventral sides and double-contoured translucent shells folded at one end. Smear usually shows acute inflammation.

Chaetomium: dematiaceous fungus that is widely encountered in soil and degrading plant material. The hyphal structures are characteristically septate, long, somewhat broad, and regular, measuring approx 4 μm in diameter and show no branching. The spores (ascospores) are usually numerous, lemon-shaped, a homogenous olive-brown color, smooth walled, and measure 8×10 μm in size. In rare cases of immunocompromised individuals, Chaetomium species can cause systemic and invasive infections with a fatal outcome (Fig. 18.5).

Pollen: common types show a double-layered wall and "air sacs" (Fig. 18.6).

Incidental Findings in the Pap Test

Collagen balls: usually occur in serous cavities, rare in the Pap test, consists of a three-dimensional structure with a hyalinized core and surrounded by benign-appearing cells. They may be transported via the fallopian tubes to the cervix.

From: *Fundamentals of Pap Test Cytology*
By: R. S. Hoda and S. A. Hoda © Humana Press Inc., Totowa, NJ

Psammoma bodies: calcified concentric structures. They may be associated with malignant
tumors (serous carcinomas of the ovary or the uterus) or nonneoplastic conditions, such as
endosalpingiosis or mesothelial hyperplasia (Fig. 18.7).

Hematoidin crystals: often associated with hemorrhage during pregnancy, pregnancy-like,
and postpartum states, golden in color, radially arranged fine needles forming cockleburs
or as aggregates of small irregular particles, spherules, or rhomboids (Fig. 18.8).

Curschman's spirals: morphologically identical to those seen in the sputum. They are only seen
in patients with a cervix and may form in endocervical mucus, but are of no clinical significance.

Herxheimer spirals: bundles of tonofibrils visible with an ordinary light microscope, which
appear as a twisty, intracytoplasmic eosinophilic structure (Fig. 18.9).

Other findings: dried mucus (Fig. 18.10), carpet beetle (Fig. 18.11), and ferning (Fig. 18.12).

Table 1
Common Contaminants in the Pap Test

Contaminants	Organisms that it may be mistaken for
Contraceptive gels	*Candida* spp.
Cotton fibers	Bacterial colonies
Fibrinous debris	*Leptothrix*
Hematoidin	*Nocardia*
Mucus	*Leptothrix*
Sulfonamide crystals	*Lactobacilli*
Vegetable cells	Squamous metaplasia
Other fungi	*Candida* spp.

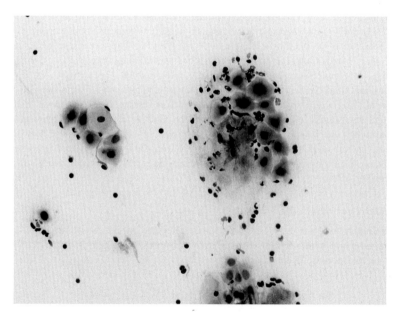

Fig. 18.1. Air-drying artifact shows cellular and nuclear enlargement with eosinophilic
staining of the nuclei (conventional smear; Papanicolaou stain).

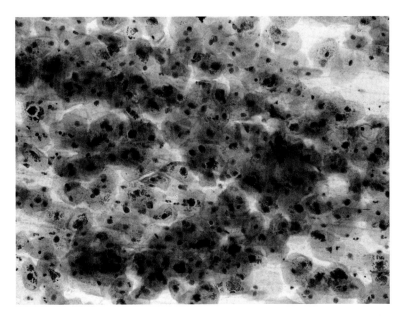

Fig. 18.2. "Corn flakes" is air trapped under a cover slip (conventional smear; Papanicolaou stain).

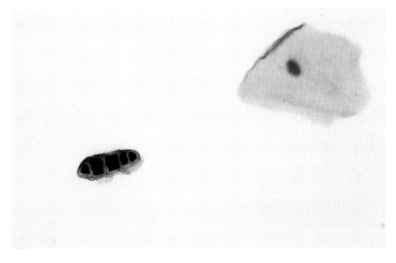

Fig. 18.3. *Alternaria*: yellow-brown pigmented structure with transverse and longitudinal septations (ThinPrep; Papanicolaou stain).

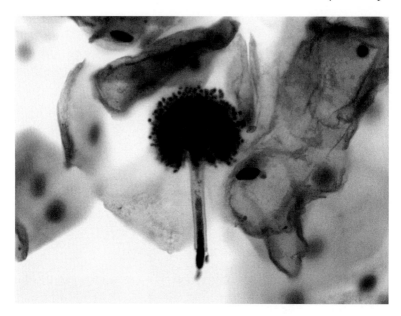

Fig. 18.4. *Aspergillus*: fruiting body comprises of a swollen vesicle at the terminus of a conidiophore, the surface of which shows one or two rows of phiallides, which in turn give rise to chains of pigmented conidia. A specialized hyphal segment, known as the foot cell, forms the base of the conidiophore (ThinPrep; Papanicolaou stain).

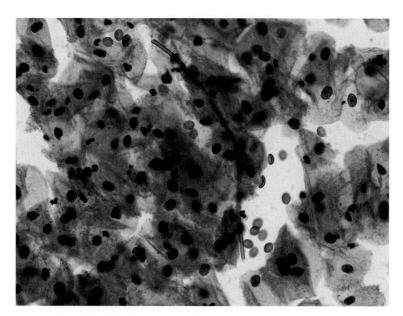

Fig. 18.5. Fungal structures consistent with *Chaetomium* spp. consist of septate and non-branching hyphae with lemon-shaped, homogenous, and olive-brown colored ascospores. It may be a contaminant or may cause fatal systemic infections in immunocompromised individuals (conventional smear; Papanicolaou stain).

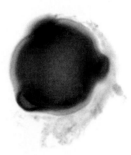

Fig. 18.6. Pollen (vegetable cells) may be a contaminant in the Pap test, especially during the summer. It is of no significance (conventional smear; Papanicolaou stain).

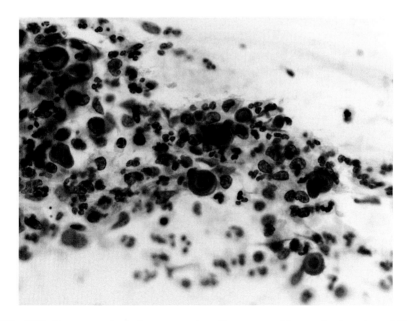

Fig. 18.7. Psammoma body in an asymptomatic woman with negative long-term follow-up (conventional smear; Papanicolaou stain).

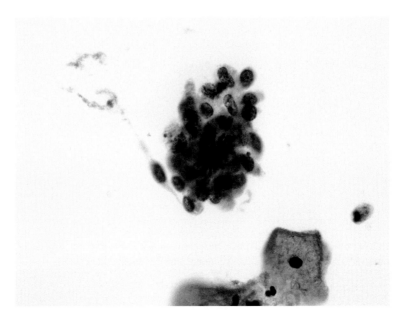

Fig. 18.8. Hematoidin crystals are golden, radially arranged needle-like structures forming cockleburs, which are rarely seen in Paps and are associated with pregnancy or the immediate postpartum period (ThinPrep; Papanicolaou stain).

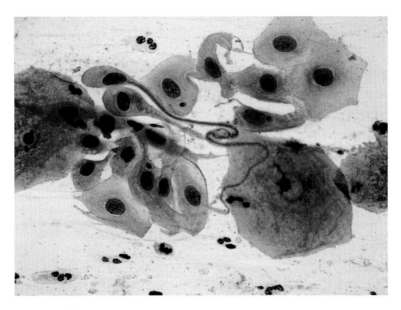

Fig. 18.9. Herxheimer's spiral: twisty intracytoplasmic eosinophic structure (conventional smear; Papanicolaou stain).

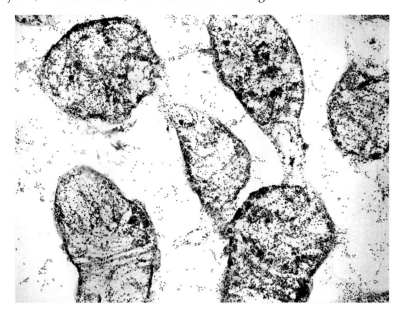

Fig. 18.10. Dried mucus in circular patches. The artifact is seen on conventional smears following radiation treatment (conventional smear; Papanicolaou stain).

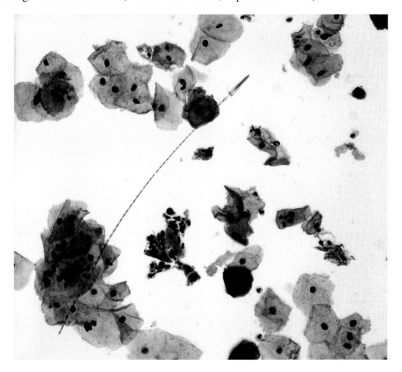

Fig. 18.11. Carpet beetle larval parts may be seen as a contaminant. The finding of the pathognomonic hastisetae (also known as "brush hair") in the smears suggests that contamination occurred at or around the time of sampling (ThinPrep; Papanicolaou stain).

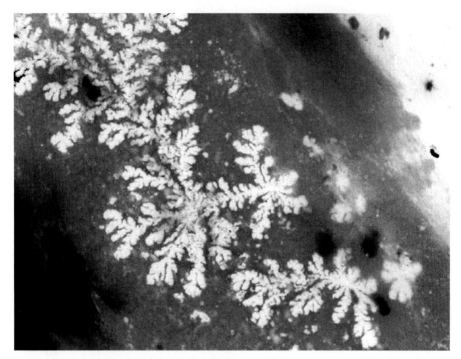

Fig. 18.12. Ferning: pattern of thin and clear cervical mucus at ovulation on a conventional smear with an air-drying artifact (conventional smear; Papanicolaou stain).

19

Screening and Management Guidelines of Pap Test and Newer Techniques

NEW CERVICAL CANCER SCREENING GUIDELINES (AMERICAN CANCER SOCIETY)

- Cervical cancer screening should begin within 3 years after the beginning of vaginal intercourse, but no later than 21 years of age.
- Cervical cancer screening should be done annually with a conventional Pap technique or every 2 years with liquid-based preparations (LBP).
- Women 30 years or older who have had three consecutive negative Pap tests may undergo testing with the Digene DNAwithPap test. If both tests are negative the woman can be screened every 2–3 years. (Please *see* Chapter 9 for more details.)
- Women 70 years of age or older who have had three consecutive negative Pap tests results and no abnormal Paps in the last 10 years may choose to stop cervical cancer screening.
- Cervical cancer screening after hysterectomy: Continued screening is not necessary in women status post-hysterectomy for benign disease and negative Pap history. Women who had a subtotal hysterectomy should continue screening at least until age 70 years. Women who had a hysterectomy for cervical precancerous lesions or cancer should continue screening.

CONSENSUS GUIDELINES FOR MANAGEMENT OF WOMEN WITH ABNORMAL PAP TEST*

P16INK4A

p16 is a cyclin-dependent kinase inhibitor that decelerates the cell cycle by inactivating the CDKs that phosphorylates the Retinoblastoma protein. p16 overexpression has been demonstrated in cervical keratinocytes, in high-grade squamous intra-epithelial lesion (HSIL) and cervical carcinoma. The overexpression of p16 results from functional inactivation of Rb by *human papillomavirus* (HPV) E7 protein. Overexpression of p16 has been shown to correlate with HPV type 16 and 18 infections and can be detected in both squamous lesions and adenocarcinomas. Because of this, p16 is emerging as a useful biomarker for HPV-induced cervical

*Figures are reproduced with permission from the American Society for Colposcopy and Cervical Pathology.

From: *Fundamentals of Pap Test Cytology*
By: R. S. Hoda and S. A. Hoda © Humana Press Inc., Totowa, NJ

Definitions of Terms Utilized in the Consensus Guidelines

Colposcopy is the examination of the cervix, vagina, and, in some instances the vulva, with the colposcope after the application of a 3-5% acetic acid solution coupled with obtaining colposcopically-directed biopsies of all lesions suspected of representing neoplasia.

Endocervical sampling includes obtaining a specimen for either histological evaluation using an endocervical curette or a cytobrush or for cytological evaluation using a cytobrush.

Endocervical assessment is the process of evaluating the endocervical canal for the presence of neoplasia using either a colposcope or endocervical sampling.

Diagnostic excisional procedure is the process of obtaining a specimen from the transformation zone and endocervical canal for histological evaluation and includes laser conization, cold-knife conization, loop electrosurgical excision (i.e., LEEP), and loop electrosurgical conization.

Satisfactory colposcopy indicates that the entire squamocolumnar junction and the margin of any visible lesion can be visualized with the colposcope.

Endometrial sampling includes obtaining a specimen for histological evaluation using an endometrial biopsy or a "dilatation and curettage" or hysteroscopy.

2002, Copyright American Society for Colposcopy and Cervical Pathology

Management of Women with Atypical Squamous Cells of Undetermined Significance (ASC-US)

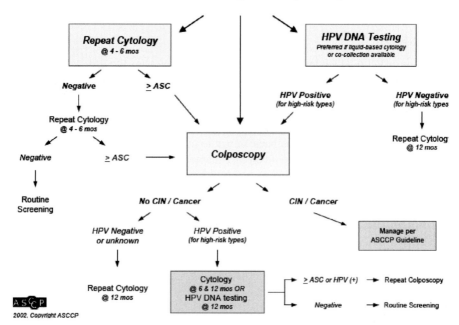

2002, Copyright ASCCP

Management of Women with Atypical Squamous Cells of Undetermined Significance (ASC-US) In Special Circumstances

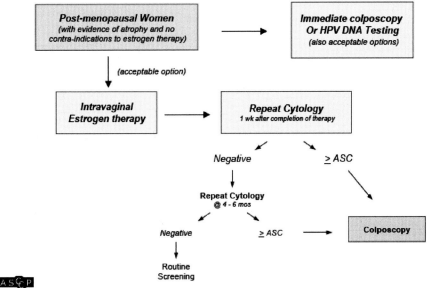

2002, Copyright American Society for Colposcopy and Cervical Pathology

Management of Women with Atypical Squamous Cells: Cannot Exclude High-grade SIL (ASC - H)

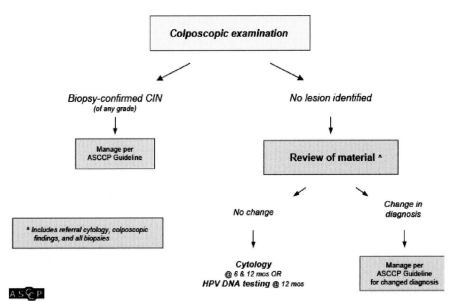

2002, Copyright American Society for Colposcopy and Cervical Pathology

Management of Women with Atypical Glandular Cells (AGC)

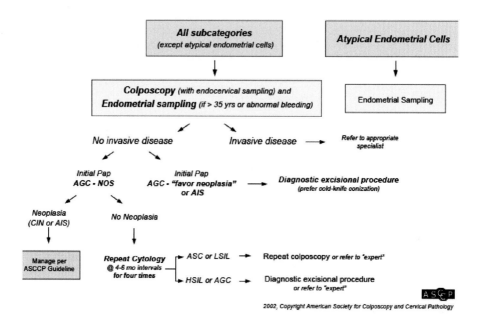

2002, Copyright American Society for Colposcopy and Cervical Pathology

Management of Women with Low-grade Squamous Intraepithelial Lesions (LSIL) *

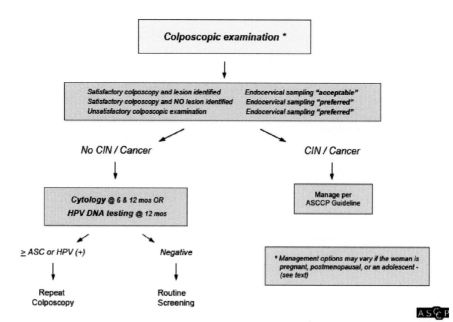

2002, Copyright American Society for Colposcopy and Cervical Pathology

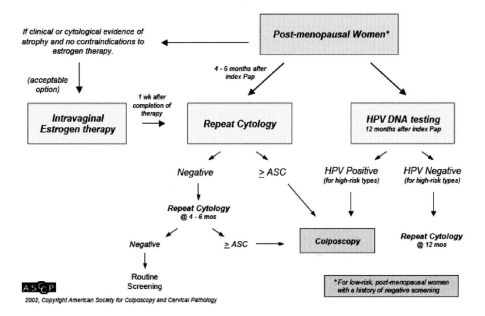

**Management of Women with Low-grade Squamous Intraepithelial Lesions
In Special Circumstances**

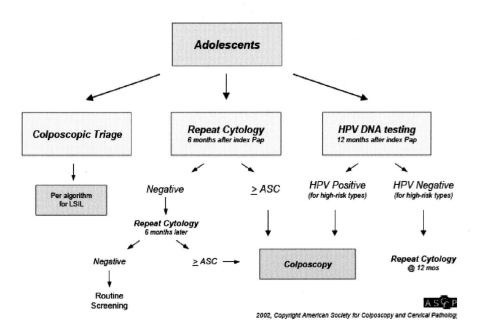

**Management of Women with Low-grade Squamous Intraepithelial Lesions
In Special Circumstances**

Management of Women with Biopsy-confirmed Cervical Intraepithelial Neoplasia - Grade 1 (CIN 1) and Satisfactory Colposcopy

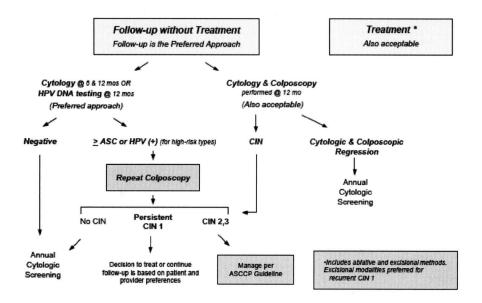

Management of Women with Biopsy-confirmed Cervical Intraepithelial Neoplasia Grade 1 (CIN 1) and Unsatisfactory Colposcopy

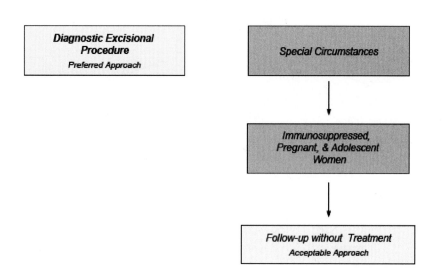

Management of Women with High-grade Squamous Intraepithelial Lesions (HSIL) *

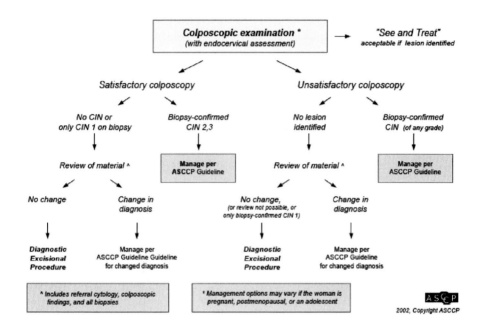

Management of Women with Biopsy-confirmed Cervical Intraepithelial Neoplasia - Grade 2 and 3 (CIN 2,3) *

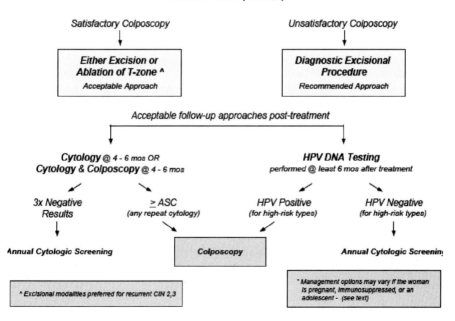

dysplastic lesions. p16INK4a protein can be immunocytochemically detected in LBP. The specificity of p16 overexpression has been examined and is associated not only with carcinoma, but also with biopsy-proven HSIL+ lesions and a significant number of cervical intra-epithelial neoplasia 1 (low-grade squamous intra-epithelial lesion, mild dysplasia) lesions.

Clinical Utility of p16

- p16 positivity may confirm the suspicion of an underlying HSIL in Paps reported as atypical squamous cells cannot exclude HSIL.
- p16 positivity may be useful in further triage of atypical squamous cells of undetermined significance or low-grade squamous intra-epithelial lesion cases that are considered "gray areas" in cervical cancer screening.
- It is convenient and cost effective.

Characteristics of p16 Detection of Squamous Intra-Epithelial Lesion

- **Sensitivity:** For detection of HSIL is 70–100%.
- **Specificity:** For detection of HSIL is 25–75%.
- **Scoring criteria for positive results:** Variable; most use a minimum of 10 positive cells per slide.
- **Staining localization:** Overexpression in both the nucleus and the cytoplasm.
- **Staining characteristics:** Diffuse and strong in lesions caused by high-risk HPV and focal and weak in lesions caused by low-risk HPV.
- **False-positive staining:** *Trichomonas vaginalis* has been reported to be positive for p16 and may be misinterpreted as dysplastic cells.

INFORM(R)® HPV ANALYTE-SPECIFIC REAGENT ASSAY

The INFORM(R) HPV analyte-specific reagent assay is a recent addition to the menu available for HPV DNA detection. INFORM HPV analyte-specific reagent assay is commercially available and is a slide-based application for HPV DNA detection that allows physicians to see the cells in their cellular context on a slide. The assay is applicable to histology, LBP (ThinPrep and SurePath) or conventional Pap slides that are incubated with fluorescein-tagged DNA probes and counter-stained. Microscopic observation of specifically stained target cells indicates HPV is present. Staining is performed on an automated instrument, the Ventana BenchMark. There are separate probe kits for oncogenic and nononcogenic HPV types. Please also *see* Chapter 9.

NOTE

The consensus Guidelines algorithms that appear in this chapter originally appeared in and are reprinted from *The Journal of Lower Genital Tract Disease*, vol. 6, issue 2, and are reprinted with the permission of ASCCP. American Society for Colposcopy and Cervical Pathology 2002. No copies of the algorithms may be made without the prior consent of ASCCP.

Appendices

Appendix 1
The Cells of the Pap Test
An Overview

From: *Fundamentals of Pap Test Cytology*
By: R. S. Hoda and S. A. Hoda © Humana Press Inc., Totowa, NJ

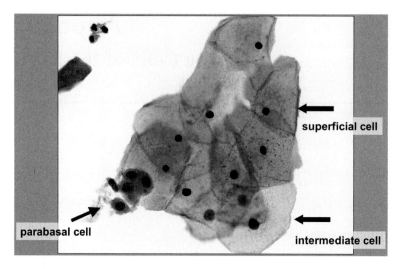

Fig. 1. Normal squamous cells in Pap smear: Superficial cells are flattened, have abundant eosinophilic cytoplasm with a transparent quality, and pyknotic nuclei. **Intermediate cells** are folded, have less abundant cyanophilic or eosinophilic cytoplasm, and vesicular nuclei; nuclear-to-cytoplasmic (n:c) ratio is lower than that of parabasal cells. **Normal parabasal cells** are round-to-oval cells with dense basophilic cytoplasms and regular nuclei and are difficult to distinguish from squamous metaplastic cells (liquid-based ThinPrep; Papanicolaou stain).

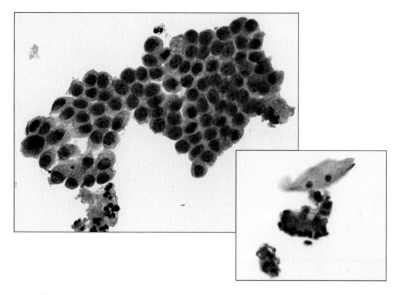

Fig. 2. Normal endocervical cells: Appear *en face* as flattened honeycombed sheets of cells with finely vacuolated cytoplasm, round nuclei, and small nucleoli. On-edge the cells are columnar with basal, ovoid nuclei (liquid-based ThinPrep; Papanicolaou stain).

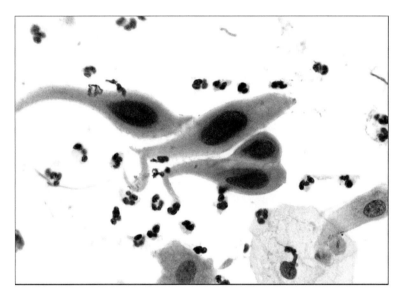

Fig. 3. Squamous metaplasia: Parabasal-type cells with variable shape, distinct cell borders, dense cytoplasm with cytoplasmic extensions, and rounded normochromic, regular nuclei with a relative increase in n:c (ThinPrep; Papanicolaou stain).

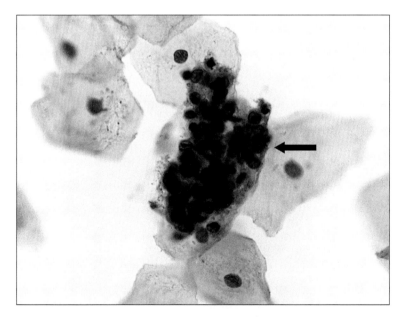

Fig. 4. Normal endometrial cells: Three-dimensional (3D) cluster of cells; nuclear size is comparable to intermediate cell nuclei and cytoplasm is scant (ThinPrep; Papanicolaou stain).

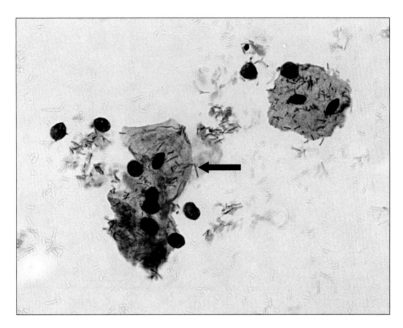

Fig. 5. *Lactobacilli:* Normal, rod-like organisms of the vaginal flora that maintain vaginal pH and produce cytolysis. "Bare" intermediate cell nuclei are seen (ThinPrep; Papanicolaou stain).

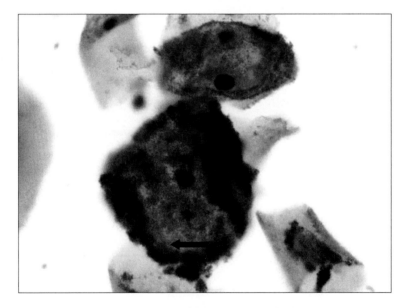

Fig. 6. "Clue" cells: Characteristic of bacterial vaginosis. Numerous small basophilic coccobacillary organisms cover the squamous cell surface (ThinPrep; Papanicolaou stain).

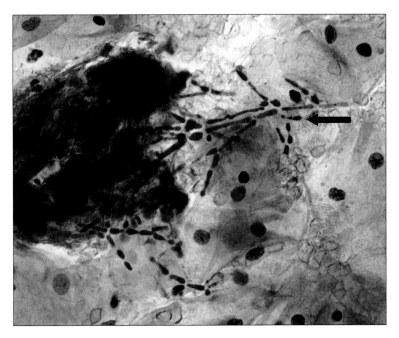

Fig. 7. *Candida albicans:* Shown with a shish-kebab effect. Mucus strands may mimic fungal organisms (ThinPrep; Papanicolaou stain).

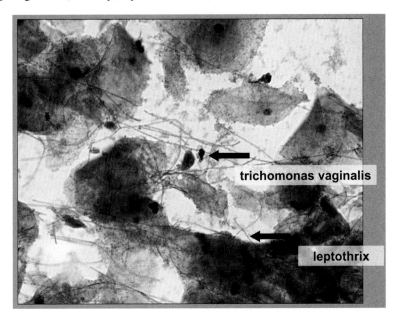

Fig. 8. *Lepthotrix:* Hair-like organisms commonly associated with *Trichomonas vaginalis* (ThinPrep; Papanicolaou stain).

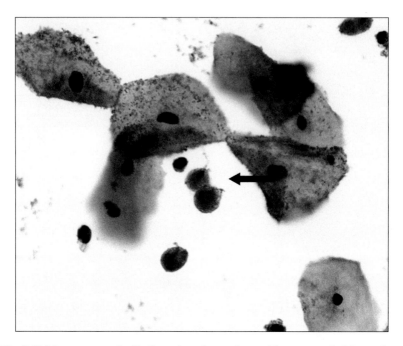

Fig. 9. *Trichomonas vaginalis:* Pear-shaped organisms with an eccentric faint nucleus and cytoplasmic granules. Differential diagnosis includes degenerated nuclei and cytoplasmic debris (ThinPrep; Papanicolaou stain).

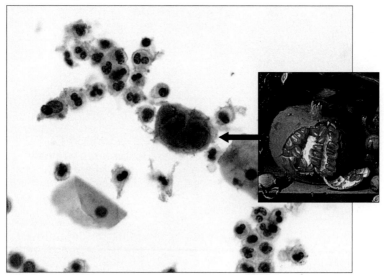

Fig. 10. Herpes simplex virus: Multinucleate giant cell with homogenous, "ground-glass" appearance of nuclei with margination of chromatin. Note nuclear molding. This infection is considered a medical emergency in pregnant patients (ThinPrep; Papanicolaou stain).

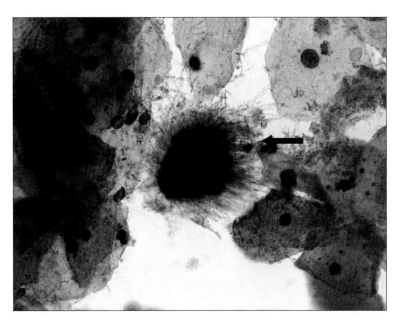

Fig. 11. *Actinomyces:* Associated with intrauterine device use. Filamentous organisms with clubbed peripheral ends are termed "Gupta bodies" (ThinPrep; Papanicolaou stain).

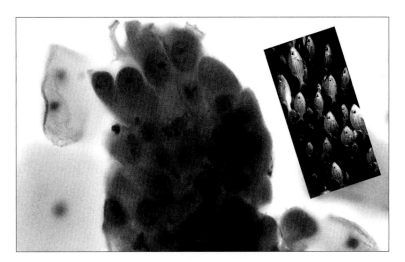

Fig. 12. Reactive/repairative squamous cells in Pap smear: May be seen in an inflammatory condition and are arranged in flat, cohesive sheets with a "streaming" effect (single cells are not seen), uniform slightly enlarged nuclei, a perinuclear halo, and small nucleoli. Repair may mimic nonkeartinizing squamous-cell carcinoma (ThinPrep; Papanicolaou stain).

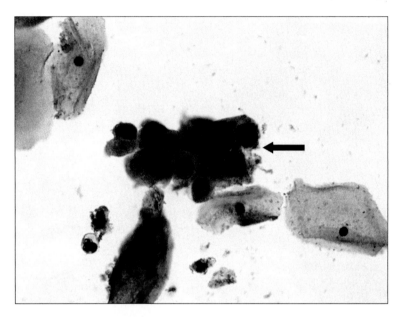

Fig. 13. Reactive endocervical cells: Are in a honeycombed sheet with slight overlap, enlarged hyperchromatic nuclei, and prominent nucleoli (ThinPrep; Papanicolaou stain).

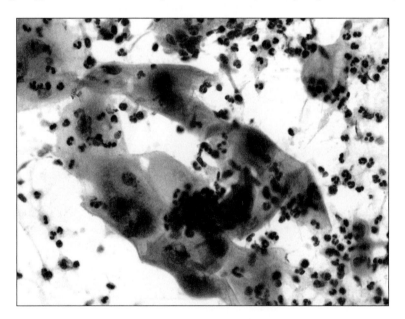

Fig. 14. Radiation change: Involves squamous and glandular cells, show enlarged cells with large nuclei, prominent nucleoli, abundant cytoplasm, nuclear and cytoplasmic vacuolation, multinucleation, intracytoplasmic inflammatory cells, and low n:c (conventional smear; Papanicolaou stain).

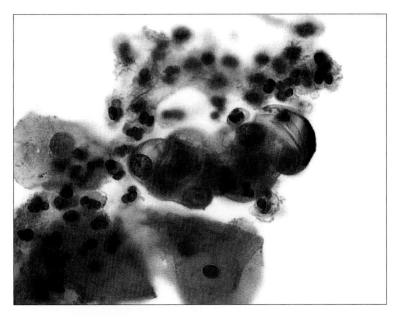

Fig. 15. Intrauterine contraceptive device cells: Are of endometrial origin. These cells appear singly with a high n:c ratio, nuclei may show atypia, and the cytoplasm is finely vacuolated (conventional smear; Papanicolaou stain).

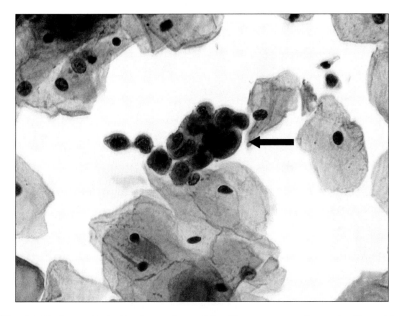

Fig. 16. Endometriosis: Benign endometrial cells are present. Stromal cells and hemosiderin may also be seen (ThinPrep; Papanicolaou stain).

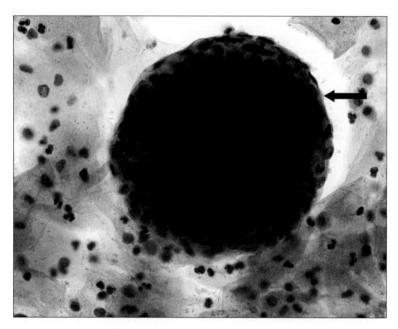

Fig. 17. "Exodus" (menstrual endometrium): Cluster of endometrial cells seen toward the end of menstruation and is comprised of glandular cells (at the periphery) and stromal cells (at the center) (ThinPrep; Papanicolaou stain).

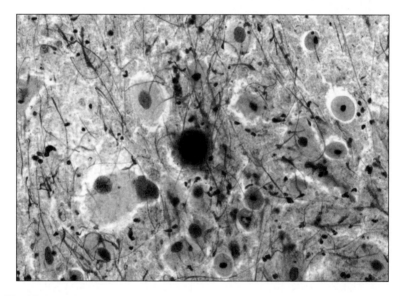

Fig. 18. Atrophy: Flat sheet of basal and parabasal cell (ThinPrep; Papanicolaou stain).

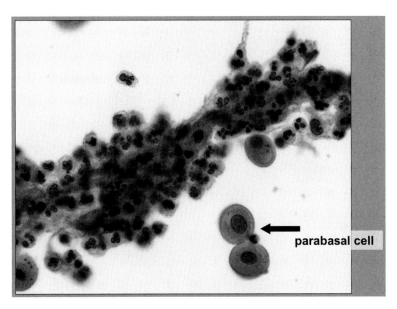

Fig. 19. Atrophic vaginitis: Parabasal cells associated with numerous inflammatory cells, mummified parabasal cells "blue-blobs," and granular background debris. The background debris is similar to tumor diathesis in squamous-cell carcinoma (conventional smear and ThinPrep; Papanicolaou stain).

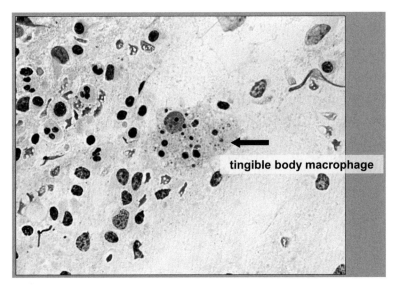

Fig. 20. Follicular cervicitis: Polymorphous lymphoid cells and tingible-body macrophages—such changes may be associated with chlamydial infection or may be misinterpreted as malignant lymphoma or high-grade squamous intra-epithelial lesion (ThinPrep; Papanicolaou stain).

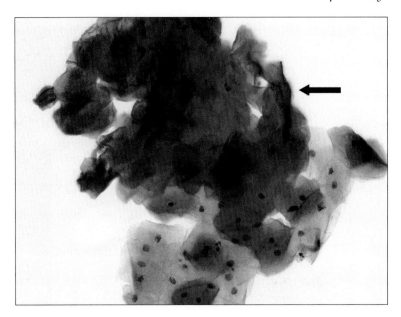

Fig. 21. Hyperkeratosis: Seen as a plaque of anucleate squames in a mucosal surface reaction in response to irritation. Although hyperkeratosis does not signify a squamous intra-epithelial lesion, it should be documented in the report, especially if extensive (HSIL) (ThinPrep; Papanicolaou stain).

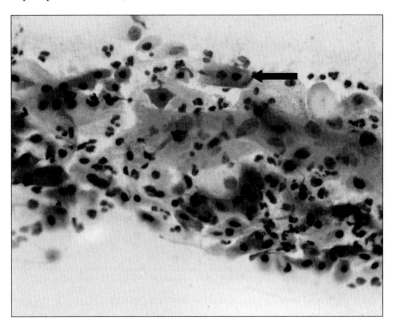

Fig. 22. Parakeratosis: Another mucosal surface reaction characterized by the presence of miniature squamous cells. These cells exfoliate either singly or in aggregates (ThinPrep; Papanicolaou stain).

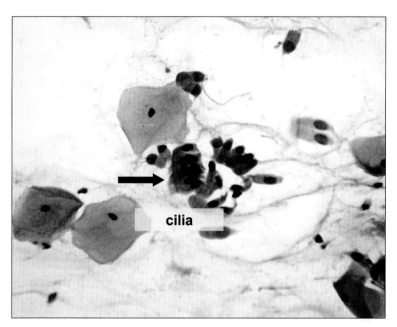

Fig. 23. Tubal metaplasia: Small strips of endocervical cells with cilia, terminal bars, and nuclear pseudostratification. It may originate from the upper endocervical canal, or may be misinterpreted as atypical glandular cells when cilia are lost during processing (conventional smear; Papanicolaou stain).

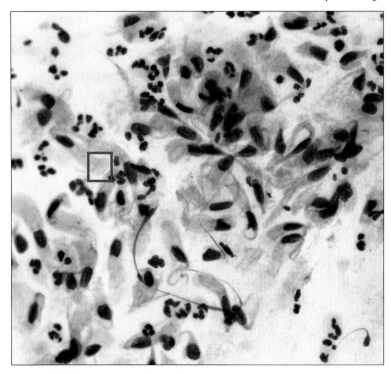

Fig. 24. Endocervical polyp: Numerous columnar endocervical cells with tubal metaplasia and spindled stromal cells may show slight nuclear atypia and may mimic adenocarcinoma *in situ* (AIS) (ThinPrep; Papanicolaou stain).

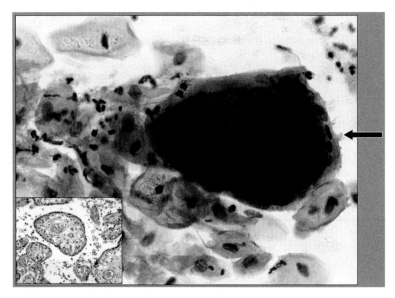

Fig. 25. Syncytiotrophoblast: Multinucleated giant cells usually seen in a postpartum smear, and may be mistaken for a high-grade malignancy (ThinPrep; Papanicolaou stain).

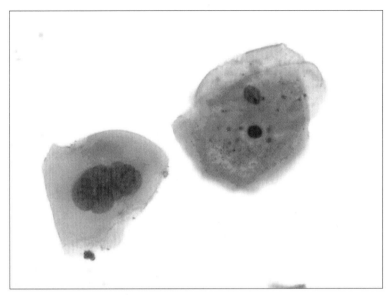

Fig. 26. Atypical squamous cells of undetermined significance: Mature cells with moderately enlarged nuclei (2.5–3 times the size of normal intermediate cell nuclei), minimal hyperchromasia, nuclear membrane irregularities, binucleation, and a mild increase in n:c. Atypical squamous cells of undetermined significance is distinguished from low-grade squamous intra-epithelial lesion (LSIL) on the basis of quality or quantity of cellular and nuclear changes (ThinPrep; Papanicolaou stain).

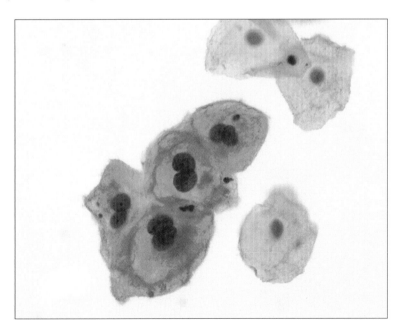

Fig. 27. Low-grade squamous intra-epithelial lesion (LSIL). Please *see* legends to **Figs. 28** and **24**.

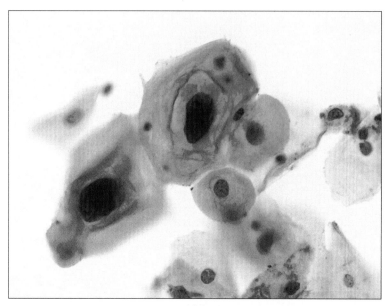

Fig. 28. LSIL (human papillomavirus [HPV] effect): Mature squamous cells with HPV effects—enlarged hyperchromatic nuclei with irregular envelope ("raisonoid") and binucleation. Cytoplasm has a sharply demarcated optically clear cytoplasmic (koilocytotic) cavity (ThinPrep; Papanicolaou stain).

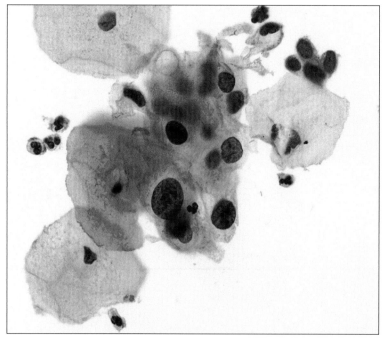

Fig. 29. LSIL (mild dysplasia): Nuclei are enlarged (more than three times the size of normal intermediate cell nuclei), hyperchromatic with mild nuclear membrane irregularity, and "mature" cytoplasm (ThinPrep; Papanicolaou stain).

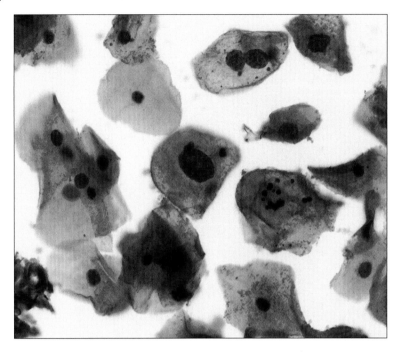

Fig. 30. LSIL. Please *see* legend to **Fig. 29** (ThinPrep; papanicolaou stain).

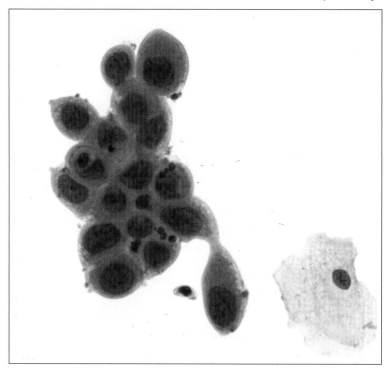

Fig. 31. Atypical squamous cells cannot exclude HSIL: Cells are of immature squamous metaplastic type. Nuclei are enlarged with slight membrane irregularity and hyperchromatic, finely granular chromatin. The n:c is not as high as HSIL (ThinPrep; Papanicolaou stain).

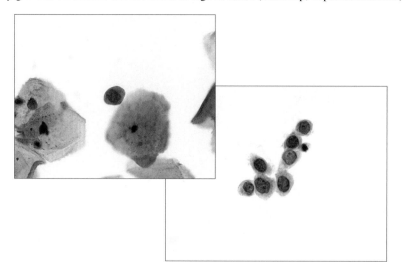

Fig. 32. HSIL: Parabasal- and metaplastic-type cells with high n:c and enlarged, hyperchromatic nuclei with marked nuclear membrane irregularity. The cytoplasm may be lacy or metaplastic in nature (ThinPrep; Papanicolaou stain).

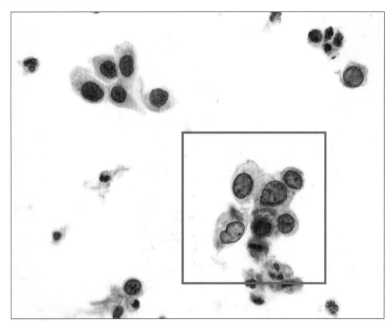

Fig. 33. HSIL. Please *see* legend to **Fig. 32** (ThinPrep; Papanicolaou stain).

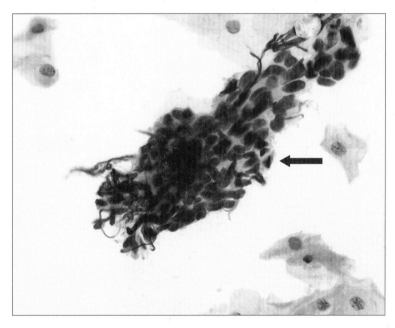

Fig. 34. HSIL involving endocervical glands: Large syncytial aggregate (ill-defined cell borders) with loss of nuclear polarity. This may be misinterpreted as atypical glandular cells and is distinguished from it by lack of "feathering" and peripheral flattening of nuclei (ThinPrep; Papanicolaou stain).

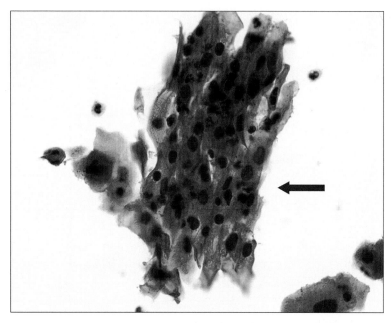

Fig. 35. Atypical parakeratosis: Sheet of elongated miniature squamous cells with atypical nuclei, cytoplasm is eosinophilic to orangeophilic, and they may be associated with LSIL (ThinPrep; Papanicolaou stain).

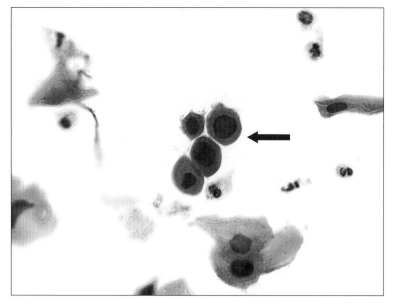

Fig. 36. Keratinizing dysplasia: Shows both nuclear and cytoplasmic pleomorphism. Note the orange cytoplasm and large hyperchromatic nuclei (ThinPrep; Papanicolaou stain).

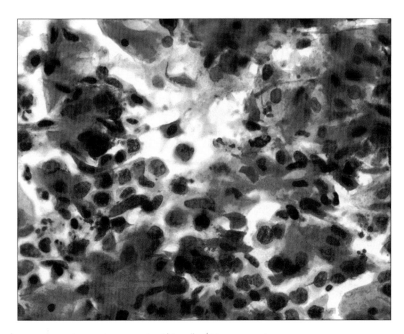

Fig. 37. Keratinizing squamous-cell carcinoma: Dispersed cells of spindle to elongated and caudate forms with heavily keratinized cytoplasm. Nuclei are pleomorphic and hyperchromatic, nucleoli are less conspicuous than the nonkeratinizing type, and tumor diathesis is generally lacking (conventional smear; Papanicolaou stain).

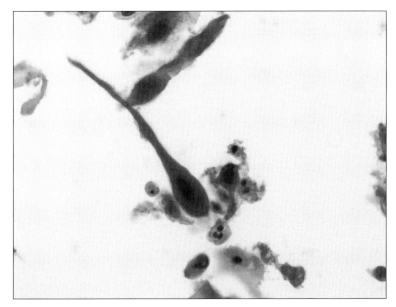

Fig. 38. Keratinizing squamous cell carcinoma. Please *see* legend to **Fig. 37.**

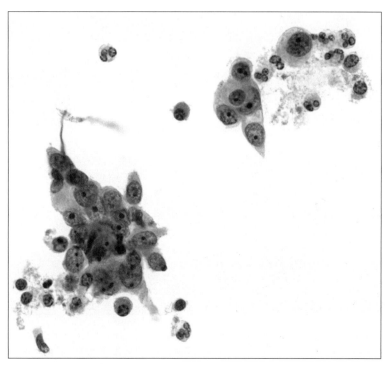

Fig. 39. Nonkeratinizing squamous-cell carcinoma: Malignant polygonal cells are arranged in either loose clusters, crowded groups, or singly. Nuclei are large, mostly round, and have coarse chromatin and macronucleoli. Cytoplasm is dense with distinct cell borders and high n:c. Tumor diathesis is generally present (ThinPrep; Papanicolaou stain).

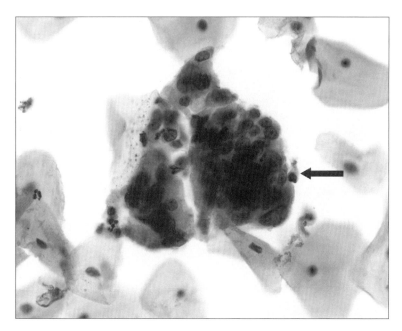

Fig. 40. Atypical glandular cells: Overcrowded cluster of glandular cells showing large, variable and hyperchromatic nuclei with small nucleoli and scant cytoplasm (ThinPrep; Papanicolaou stain).

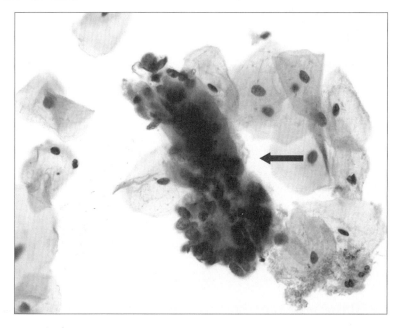

Fig. 41. Atypical endocervical cells: Two-dimensional sheet with focal palisading, "pseudo-feathering," hyperchromatic nuclei, and nucleoli may be present (ThinPrep; Papanicolaou stain).

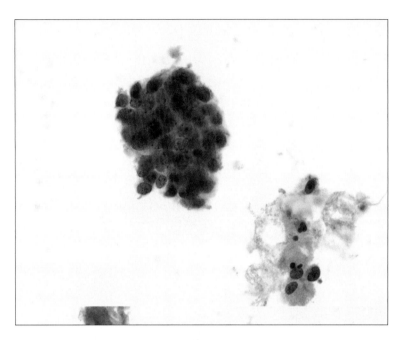

Fig. 42. Atypical endometrial cells: 3D cluster of cells with hyperchromatic nuclei, nucleoli, and scanty cytoplasm (ThinPrep; Papanicolaou stain).

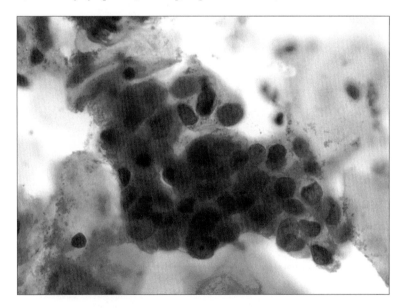

Fig. 43. Atypical endocervical cells, favor neoplastic: Crowded sheet of atypical endocervical cells with nuclear overlap and focal "feathering" (ThinPrep and conventional smear; Papanicolaou stain).

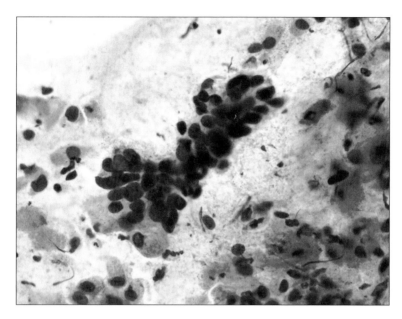

Fig. 44. Endocervical AIS: "feathering" is the classic pattern of AIS and elongated hyperchromatic nuclei (ThinPrep; Papanicolaou stain).

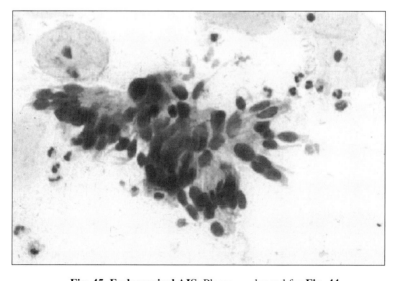

Fig. 45. Endocervical AIS. Please *see* legend for **Fig. 44**.

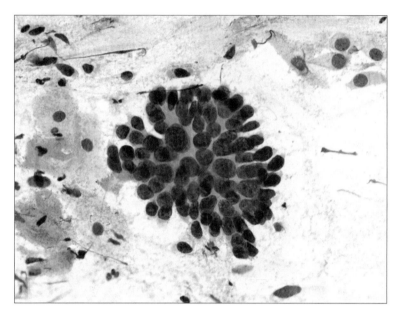

Fig. 46. Endocervical AIS. Please *see* legend to **Figs. 44** and **45** (conventional smear; papanicolaou stain).

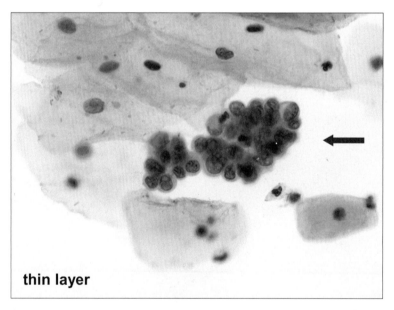

thin layer

Fig. 47. Endometrial adenocarcinoma: 3D cluster with hyperchromatic nuclei, nucleoli, watery diathesis, and intracytoplasmic neutrophils (ThinPrep and conventional smear; Papanicolaou stain).

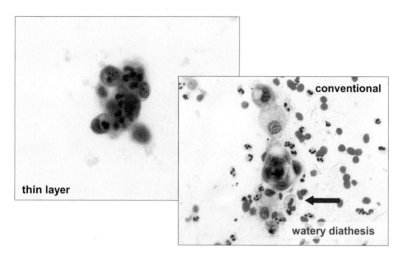

Fig. 48. Endometrial adenocarcinoma. Please *see* legend to **Fig. 47** (Papanicolaou stain).

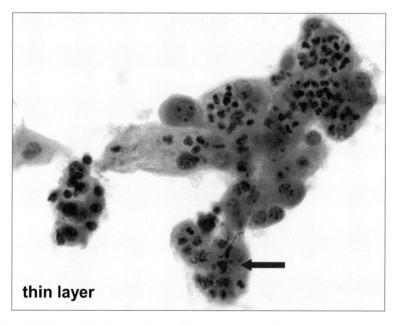

Fig. 49. Endometrial adenocarcinoma. Please *see* legend to **Fig. 47** (ThinPrep; Papanicolaou stain).

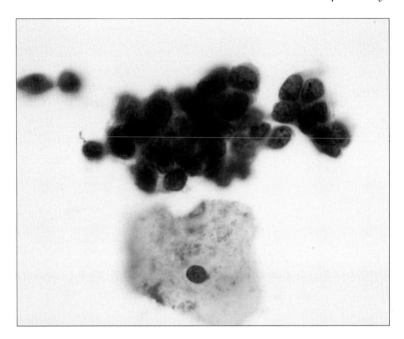

Fig. 50. Small-cell carcinoma of cervix: Shows aggregate of small irregular tumor cells with scant cytoplasm and small nuclei. Nuclear molding is seen (ThinPrep; Papanicolaou stain).

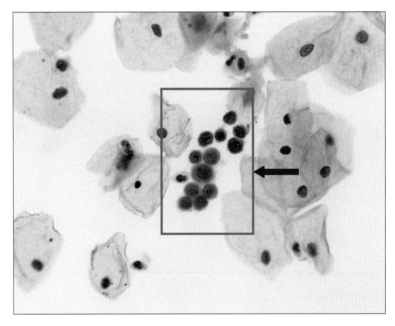

Fig. 51. Metastatic lobular carcinoma of breast: Shows a cluster of small cells with large irregular nuclei and scant cytoplasm. Clean background of the smear is often observed in metastatic tumors. Clinical history is of extrauterine malignancy is important (ThinPrep; Papanicolaou stain).

Appendix 2
Suggested Readings

1. Wright TC Jr, Cox JT, Massad LS, et al. 2001 consensus guidelines for management of women with cervical squamous intraepithelial neoplasia. Am J Obstet Gynecol, 2003;189:295–304.
2. Acs G, Gupta PK, Baloch ZW. Glandular and squamous atypia and intraepithelial lesions in atrophic cervicovaginal smears. Acta Cytol 2000;44:611–617.
3. al-Nafussi A, Rebello G, al-Yusif R, et al. The borderline cervical smear: colposcopic and biopsy outcome. J Clin Pathol 2000;53:439–444.
4. Baker JJ. Conventional and liquid-based cervicovaginal cytology: A comparison study with clinical and histologic follow-up. *Diagn Cytopathol* 2002;27:185–188.
5. Bergeron C, Bishop J, Lemarie A, et al. Accuracy of thin-layer cytology in patients undergoing cervical cone biopsy. Acta Cytol 2001;45:519–524.
6. Biscotti CV, O'Brien DL, Gero MA, et al. Thin-layer Pap test vs. conventional Pap smear. Analysis of 400 split samples. J Reprod Med 2002;47:9–13.
7. Brogi E, Tambouret R, Bell DA. Classification of benign endometrial glandular cells in cervical smears from postmenopausal women. Cancer 2002;96:60–66.
8. Bulten J, de Wilde PC, Boonstra H, et al. Proliferation in "atypical" atrophic pap smears. Gynecol Oncol 2000;79:225–229.
9. Cenci M, Vecchione A. Atypical squamous and glandular cells of undetermined significance (ASCUS and AGUS) of the uterine cervix. Anticancer Res 2000;20:3701–3707.
10. Chhieng DC, Elgert P, Cohen JM, et al. Clinical implications of atypical glandular cells of undetermined significance, favor endometrial origin. Cancer 2001;93:351–356.
11. Cox JT. American Society for Colposcopy and Cervical Pathology. The clinician's view: role of human papillomavirus testing in the American Society for Colposcopy and Cervical Pathology Guidelines for the management of abnormal cervical cytology and cervical cancer precursors. Arch Pathol Lab Med 2003;127:950.
12. Cuzick, J. et al. Management of women who test positive for high–risk types of human papillomavirus: the HART study. The Lancet 2003;362:1871–1876.
13. DeMay RM. Hyperchromatic crowded groups: pitfalls in pap smear diagnosis. Am J Clin Pathol 2000;114 Suppl:S36–S43.
14. DeMay RM. Should we abandon Pap smear testing? Am J Clin Pathol 2000;114 Suppl:S48–S51.
15. DeMay RM. Common problems in Papanicolaou smear interpretation. Arch Pathol Lab Med 1997; 121:229.
16. Demirezen S. Pinus pollen in a vaginal smear. Acta Cytol 2000;44:481–482.
17. Demirezen S. Review of cytologic criteria of bacterial vaginosis: examination of 2,841 Papanicolaou-stained vaginal smears. Diagn Cytopathol 2003;29:156–159.
18. Fadare O, Chacho MS, Parkash V. Psammoma bodies in cervicovaginal smears: significance and practical implications for diagnostic cytopathology. Adv Anat Pathol 2004;11:250–261.
19. Finan RR, Irani-Hakime N, Tamim H, et al. Detection of human papillomavirus (HPV) genotypes in cervico-vaginal scrapes of women with normal and abnormal cytology. Clin Microbiol Infect. 2001;7:688–692.
20. Fredricks DN, Fiedler TL, Marrazzo JM. Molecular identification of bacteria associated with bacterial vaginosis. N Engl J Med 2005;353:1899–1911.

From: *Fundamentals of Pap Test Cytology*
By: R. S. Hoda and S. A. Hoda © Humana Press Inc., Totowa, NJ

21. Green KM, Turyan HV, Hoda RS, et al. Metastatic lobular carcinoma in a ThinPrep Pap test: Cytomorphology and differential diagnosis. Diagn Cytopathol 2005;33:58–59.
22. Gupta D, Balsara G. Extrauterine malignancies. Role of Pap smears in diagnosis and management. Acta Cytol 1999;43:806–813.
23. Hecht JL, Sheets EE, Lee KR. Atypical glandular cells of undetermined significance in conventional cervical/vaginal smears and thin-layer preparations. *Cancer* 2002;25;96:1–4.
24. Hoda SA, Hoda RS. "Chewing gum" and "corn flakes": similes in cytopathology. Diagn Cytopathol 1994;10:397.
25. Hoda RS, Hoda SA. "Orphan Annie" nuclei and "strawberry gall bladders": Modern Pathology 1993;6:637–638.
26. Hoda RS. "Mercury drops" and "spider legs": Yet more similes in cytopathology. Diagn Cytopathol 1995;13:368.
27. Hoda RS, Hoda SA. Yet more analogies in cytopathology. Diagn Cytopathol 2004;30:133.
28. Hoda RS, Colello C, Roddy M, Houser PM. "Fruiting body" of Aspergillus species in a routine cervico-vaginal smear (Pap test). Diagn Cytopathol 2005;33:244–245.
29. Hoda RS, Parrett T, Madory J, Jones JB, Zhang D, Minamiguchi S. Metastatic Merkel cell carcinoma in a Pap smear. Acta Cytologica 2004;48:586–588.
30. Irvin W, Evans SR, Andersen W, et al. The utility of HPV DNA triage in the management of cytological AGC. Am J Obstet Gynecol 2005;193:559–565.
31. Keating JT, Wang HH. Significance of a diagnosis of atypical squamous cells of undetermined significance for Papanicolaou smears in perimenopausal and postmenopausal women. Cancer 2001;93:100–105.
32. Klinkhamer PJ, Meerding WJ, Rosier PF, Hanselaar AG. Liquid-based cervical cytology. Cancer 2003;99:263–271.
33. Koss LG, Melamed MR. Koss' Diagnostic Cytology and Its Histopathologic Bases, 5th ed. Philadelphia: Lippincott; 2005.
34. Laudadio J, Hoda RS. Unique appearance of *Actinomyces* on ThinPrep Pap test Actinomyces in ThinPrep. Diagn Cytopathol 2006;34:553.
35. Levine PH, Waisman J, Mittal K. Significance of the cytologic diagnosis of endocervical glandular involvement in high-grade squamous intraepithelial lesions. Diagn Cytopathol 2002;26:217–221.
36. Lorincz A, Richart R. Human Papillomavirus DNA testing as an adjunct to cytology in cervical screening programs. APLM 2003;127:959–968.
37. Luzzatto R, Poli M, Recktenvald M, et al. Human papillomavirus infection in atrophic smears.A case report. Acta Cytol 2000;44:420–422.
38. Llewellyn H. Observer variation, dysplasia grading, and HPV typing: a review. Am J Clin Pathol 2000;114 Suppl:S21–S35.
39. Martinez-Giron R, Ribas-Barcelo A. Algae in cytologic smears. Acta Cytol 2001;45:936–940.
40. Martinez-Giron R, Gonzalez-Lopez JR, Escobar-Stein J., et al. Freshwater microorganisms and other arthropods in Papanicolaou smears. Diagn Cytopathol 2005;32:222–225.
41. Martin-Hirsch PL, Koliopoulos G, Paraskevaidis E. Is it now time to evaluate the true accuracy of cervical cytology screening? A review of the literature. Eur J Gynaecol Oncol 2002;23:363–365.
42. Mathers ME, Johnson SJ, Wadehra V. How predictive is a cervical smear suggesting glandular neoplasia? Cytopathology 2002;13:83–91.
43. Mattosinho de Castro Ferraz Mda G, Focchi J, Stavale JN, Nicolau SM, Rodrigues de Lima G, Baracat EC. Atypical glandular cells of undetermined significance. Cytologic predictive value for glandular involvement in high grade squamous intraepithelial lesions. Acta Cytol 2003;47:154–158.
44. MGrath CM, Kurtis JD, Yu GH. Evaluation of mild to moderate dysplasia on cervical endocervical Pap smear: a subgroup of patients who bridge LSIL and HSIL. Diagn Cytopathol 2000;23:245–248.
45. Migliore G, Rossi E, Aldovini A, et al. Variation in the assessment of adequacy in cervical smears. Cytopathology 2001;12:377–382.
46. Morrison C, Prokorym P, Piquero C, et al. Oral contraceptive pills are associated with artifacts in ThinPrep Pap smears that mimic low-grade squamous intraepithelial lesions. Cancer 2003;25;99:75–82.

47. Nygard JF, Sauer T, Skjeldestad FE, Skare GB, Thoresen SO. CIN 2/3 and cervical cancer after an ASCUS pap smear. A 7-year, prospective study of the Norwegian population-based, coordinated screening program. Acta Cytol 2003;47:991–1000.
48. Nasser SM, Cibas ES, Crum C. The significance of low-grade squamous intraepithelial lesion cannot exclude high-grade squamous intraepithelial lesion. Cancer Cytopathol 2003;99: 272–276.
49. Nasuti JF, Fleisher SR, Gupta PK. Atypical glandular cells of undetermined significance (AGUS): clinical considerations and cytohistologic correlation. Diagn Cytopathol 2002;26:186–190.
50. O'Meara A. Present standards for cervical cancer screening. Curr Opin Oncol 2002;14:505–511.
51. Okuyama T, Maeda S, Kobayashi TK, Takahashi R. Detection of Trichomonas vaginalis by combined A6p and P65 sequences using PCR amplification from Papanicolaou-stained smears. Acta Cytol 2003;47:696–698.
52. Oliveira ER, Derchain SF, Rabelo-Santos SH, et al. Detection of high-risk human papillomavirus (HPV) DNA by Hybrid Capture II in women referred due to atypical glandular cells in the primary screening. Diagn Cytopathol 2004;31:19–22.
53. Papanicolau Society of Cytopathology Practice Guidelines Task Force. Papanicolaou Society of Cytopathology guidelines for educational notes, disclaimers, and similar comments on reports of cervical cytology specimens. Diagn Cytopathol 2003;28:282–285.
54. Pientong C, Ekalaksananan T, Swadpanich U, Kongyingyoes B, Kritpetcharat O, Yuenyao P, Ruckait N. Immunocytochemical detection of p16INK4a protein in scraped cervical cells. Acta Cytol 2003;47:616–623.
55. Payandeh F, Koss LG. Nuclear grooves in normal and abnormal cervical smears. Acta Cytol 2003;47:421–425.
56. Rau AR, Saldanha P, Raghuveer CV, et al. Metastatic lobular mammary carcinoma diagnosed in cervicovaginal smears: A case report. Diagn Cytopathol 2003;29:300–302.
57. Renshaw AA, Dubry-Benstein B, Haja J, et al. Cytologic features of low grade squamous intraepithelial lesion in ThinPrep Papanicolaou slides and conventional smears. Arch Pathol Lab Med 2005;129:23–25.
58. Selvaggi SM, Guidos BJ. Endocervical component: is it a determinant of specimen adequacy? Diagn Cytopathol 2002;26:53–55.
59. Sherman ME, Solomon D, Schiffman M. Qualification of ASCUS. A comparison of equivocal LSIL and equivocal HSIL cervical cytology in the ASCUS LSIL Triage Study. Am J Clin Pathol 2001;116:386–394.
60. Sherman ME, et al. Human Papillomavirus testing, and risk for cervical neoplasia: a 10-year cohort analysis. J Nat Cancer Inst 2003;95:46–52.
61. Shin CH, Schorge JO, Lee KR, et al. Cytologic and biopsy findings leading to conization in adeno-carcinoma in situ of the cervix. Obstet Gynecol 2002;100:271–276.
62. Simsir A, Hwang S, Cangiarella J, et al. Glandular cell atypia on Papanicolaou smears: inter-observer variability in the diagnosis and prediction of cell of origin. Cancer 2003;99:323–330.
63. Smith JH. Bethesda 2001. Review. Cytopathology 2002;13:4–10.
64. Smith-McCune K, Mancuso V, Contant T, et al. Management of women with atypical Papanicolaou tests of undetermined significance by board-certified gynecologists: discrepancies with published guidelines. Am J Obstet Gynecol 2001;185:551–556.
65. Solomon D, et al. Comparison of three management strategies for patients with atypical squamous cells of undetermined significance: baseline results from a randomized trial, J. Nat Cancer Inst 2001;93:293–299.
66. Solomon D, Davey D, Kurman R, et al. The 2001 Bethesda System: terminology for reporting results of cervical cytology. JAMA 2002;287:2114–2119.
67. Solomon D, Schiffman M, Tarone R. ASCUS LSIL Triage Study (ALTS) conclusions reaffirmed: response to a November 2001 commentary. Obstet Gynecol 2002;99:671–674.
68. Solomon D, Davey D, Kurman R, et al. The 2001 Bethesda System: terminology for reporting results of cervical cytology. JAMA 2002;287:2114–2119.
69. Solomon D. Update on cervical screening. Gynecol oncol 2005;99(Suppl 1):S13.

70. Studeman KD, Ioffe OB, Puszkiewicz J, Sauvegeot J, Henry MR. Effect of cellularity on the sensitivity of detecting squamous lesions in liquid-based cervical cytology. Acta Cytol 2003;47:605–610.

71. Szporn A, Chen X, Wu M, et al. Collagen balls in cervica-vaginal smears. Acta Cytol. 2005;49:262–264.

72. van der Laak JA, de Bie LM, de Leeuw H, et al. The effect of Replens on vaginal cytology in the treatment of postmenopausal atrophy: cytomorphology versus computerised cytometry. J Clin Pathol 2002;55:446–451.

73. Wang N, Emancipator SN, Rose P, et al. Histologic follow-up of atypical endocervical cells. Liquid-based, thin-layerpreparation vs. conventional Pap smear. Acta Cytol 2002;46:453–457.

74. Williamson BA, DeFrias D, Gunn R, Tarjan G, Nayar R. Significance of extensive hyperkeratosis on cervical/vaginal smears. Acta Cytol 2003;47:749–752.

75. Wu HH, Schuetz MJ 3rd, Cramer H. Significance of benign endometrial cells in Pap smears from postmenopausal women. J Reprod Med 2001;46:795–798.

76. Yang YJ, Trapkin LK, Demoski RK, et al. The small blue cell dilemma associated with tamoxifen therapy. Arch Pathol Lab Med 2001;125:1047–1050.

77. Zardawi IM, Rode JW. Clinical value of repeat Pap smear at the time of colposcopy. Acta Cytol 2002;46:495–498.

78. Zardawi IM. Cellularity of liquid-based, thin-layer cervical cytology. Acta Cytol 2003;47:943.

Index

A

Abnormal Pap test
consensus guidelines for management, 187–188
Acanthosis, 1
Acidophilia, 1
Actinomyces, 1, 63t, 66, 67f, 68f, 203f
Acute radiation changes, 173
Adenocarcinoma. *See also* Endocervical adenocarcinoma;
Endometrial adenocarcinoma
metastatic serous
of endometrium, 166f
Adenocarcinoma *in situ* (AIS), 127–138
bird tail, 131f
differential diagnosis of, 132
endocervical, 123, 221f
feathering, 129f, 130f
flat sheet, 130f
vs HSIL, 107, 110f, 138t
vs LUS, 138t
vs SIL, 132t
similarities to SIL, 128
strip, 131f
vs tubal metaplasia, 137t
AGC. *See* Atypical glandular cells (AGC)
AGC-NOS. *See* Atypical glandular cells not otherwise specified (AGC-NOS)
Air-drying artifacts, 1, 179, 180f
AIS. *See* Adenocarcinoma *in situ* (AIS)
Alternaria, 1, 179
Amenorrhea, 1
American Cancer Society
new cervical cancer screening guidelines, 187
Amorphous, 1
Amphophilia, 1
Anaplasia, 1
Anisocytosis, 1

Anisokaryosis, 1
Anucleate squames, 1
Apoptosis, 1
Arias–Stella reaction, 1, 43, 46f, 160, 160f
Artifacts, 179
air-drying, 1, 179, 180f
brown, 2, 179
brush, 2
ASC. *See* Atypical squamous cells (ASC)
ASC-H. *See* Atypical squamous cells cannot exclude high-grade squamous intra-epithelial lesion (ASC-H)
ASC-US. *See* Atypical squamous cells of undetermined significance (ASC-US)
Aspergillus, 182f
Atrophic smears, 1, 40
Atrophic vaginitis, 1, 49f–51f, 207f
blue blob in, 121f, 122
vs squamous carcinoma, 42t, 120
Atrophy, 42, 47f–48f, 50f, 206f
atypical, 87, 87f, 88f
diagnostic pitfalls in, 41t
differential diagnosis of, 41t
giant histiocytic cell in, 52f
vs small-cell carcinoma, 41t
Atypia, 1
Atypical atrophy, 87, 87f, 88f
Atypical endocervical cells, 219f, 220f
Atypical endometrial cells, 220f
Atypical endometrial epithelial cells, 150
Atypical endometrial hyperplasia, 152
Atypical glandular cells (AGC), 124, 219f
endocervical lesions, 123
favor neoplastic, 126f, 127f, 128f
follow-up, 126
management of, 190